SAUNDERS MEDICAL AND NURSING DICTIONARIES
AND VOCABULARY AIDS

Dorland's Illustrated Medical Dictionary

Dorland's Pocket Medical Dictionary

Cole: The Doctor's Shorthand

Jablonski: Illustrated Dictionary of Eponymic
Syndromes and Diseases

Leader & Leader: Dictionary of Comparative
Pathology and Experimental Biology

Miller–Keane: Encyclopedia and Dictionary of
Medicine and Nursing

Sloane: The Medical Word Book — A Spelling and
Vocabulary Guide to Medical Transcription

The Doctor's Shorthand

Frank Cole, M.D.

Editor, Nebraska State Medical Journal
Clinical Associate, Department of Surgery,
University of Nebraska College of Medicine;
Consultant in Anesthesiology, Lincoln
Veterans Administration Hospital

W. B. SAUNDERS COMPANY
Philadelphia · London · Toronto

W. B. Saunders Company: West Washington Square
                          Philadelphia, Pa.   19105

                          12 Dyott Street
                          London, WC1A   1DB

                          833 Oxford Street
                          Toronto, Ontario M8Z 5T9, Canada

The Doctor's Shorthand   ISBN 0-7216-2643-2

Print No.:   9   8   7   6   5   4

For Doris, Jill, Jim, and Tom

Preface

Doctors are rugged individualists. They insist on keeping records, and they dislike keeping records. They write orders and prescriptions and certificates and progress notes. They take histories and fill out examination reports. They write illegibly, and they resort to dictation when they can. They have fled to Latin so that their foreign colleagues understand, and to keep the patient from knowing more than is good for him. But they write all day long; they write while they examine, and they write while they treat. It is no wonder, then, that they have taken refuge in hieroglyphics, in symbols, and in abbreviations. There is the apocryphal story of the doctor who could write a whole history and physical on one side of a tongue depressor. I will not quarrel with the story's authenticity. I have caught myself putting a throat stick into a patient's mouth, seeing too late that it contained similar valuable notes. Or what is worse, I have come home and searched for the notes, only to remember that I had looked into someone's pharynx and then thrown away my tongue depressor-notebook.

All of the abbreviations in this book have been seen. I did not make any of them up. They were found on charts, in medical journals, and on other doctors' tongue depressors, and they were supplied by helpful colleagues. I hope you enjoy them. In deciphering what physicians have written, I hope they will help you.

Abbreviations are efficient: they are timesaving, and particularly they are spacesaving. They have changed with the years. Our predecessors used to say things like, "Let a draught be made"; they ordered sea-water baths; and they prescribed in scruples and drachms.

I have omitted chemical symbols; everybody knows them, and you can look them up in other books, anyway. This book is to help you get through "No c/o, up ad lib, HS care, to BR: RN." It will help you to translate "ORFD, G&T." If you are an anesthesiologist, it will enable you to understand a neurosurgeon's notes, for if doctors have a written language all their own, each specialty has its very own dialect. "HD" is heart disease to the cardiologist, but it means hearing distance to his ENT friend. "MS" suggests multiple sclerosis to the neurologist, but it means morphine sulphate to the charge nurse; it stands for musculoskeletal to the intern and orthopedist, for mitral stenosis to the internist, and for manuscript to the editor.

Periods have been omitted, since they serve no useful purpose and are left out in modern medical writing and in doctors' notes. Where lower case is important, I have used it; otherwise, capital letters are used for abbreviations, to separate them from their definitions. I have attempted to avoid the acronymic horror in which the letters do not stand for the words. I have omitted many abbreviations that are not in common use; some are occasionally invented for a single journal article and are not met elsewhere.

New abbreviations appear in the literature, like arterial bleeding, in spurts; this list has been closed several times only to be reopened when a fresh burst of initials flooded the journals. It is well to point out that not all abbreviations abbreviate. Writing "@" instead of "at" saves neither time nor effort, and substituting "stat" for "now" wastes both. However, since motivation may consist of other things, even the striving for elegance, such notations do appear and therefore are included in these pages.

Some abbreviations will not be found here, for obvious reasons: The elements and most of the chemical compounds, the vitamins, pharmaceutical companies (as SKF, PD, BD, and MSD), state medical societies, components of the electrocardiogram, individual members of the ABO and Rh blood systems, and board specialties.

Abbreviation-hunting is a sport, and its devotees can become the most avid of collectors. Skimming through article after article with magnifying glass, searching for initials, these weary eyes fell upon Ecg, then Eeg, and finally on one not seen before, Egg. But it was only that most friable of articles, the egg. And one day I found EGG, too, and even MOM and POP.

The search was fun, but the collection represents more work than was anticipated. Day after day ended with PM (proofreader's myopia), when the words could no longer be read and only sleep (NREM) would prove the specific RX for my VA. Hours were spent, after seeing an abbreviation in a table, backtracking endlessly through the article to find its meaning. And too often, the initials were never defined, which is why this book was written. They were doggedly and ruthlessly hunted down, so that a future reader confronted with the same problem would know what was meant. And sometimes rereading the article revealed that the initials were an author's ("one of us") or a patient's.

But the pursuit was neither dry nor fruitless. It showed that SPCA may have nothing to do with cruelty to animals, that ABC is not the alphabet, that PTA does not always refer to teachers, and that MIT is not necessarily a school nor is HOOD a criminal. CPA may not be an accountant, and you can't eat PIE or feed a CAT. And nobody loved AMY.

Not all abbreviations consist of letters, so I have included a special section where you will find such interesting things as that a square means male, a circle mean female; a vertical arrow means decreased if it points down and increased if it's up; a circle with a horizontal line through it means, my neurosurgical friend says, "normal."

I hope this book will help both to make medical reading easier, since articles are coming to consist largely, if not entirely, of unexplained symbols (even when the article defines its shorthand, the abstract does not), and, particularly, to standardize abbreviations used in medical writing. I am indebted to all my friends who brought me their abbreviations and who listened to mine; and to those who shared with me the fun of tracking down these elusive symbols, especially when I was allowed to feel that I was doing something of any value.

Lincoln, Nebraska   FRANK COLE, M.D.

A

A	absolute temperature
	absorbence
	accommodation
	acetum
	Actinomyces
	age
	allergy
	ampere
	Angstrom unit
	anode
	Anopheles
	anterior
	artery
	atropine
	axial
	before (*ante*)
	mass number
	start of anesthesia
	total acidity
	water (*aqua*)
A₂	second aortic sound
AA	acetic acid
	achievement age
	Addicts Anonymous
	Alcoholics Anonymous
	alveolar-arterial
	aminoacetone
	arteries
	ascending aorta
	of each (*ana*)
A&A	aid and attendance
AAA	abdominal aortic aneurysm
	amalgam
	American Academy of Allergy
	androgenic anabolic agent
AAALAC	American Association for Accreditation of Laboratory Animal Care
AAAM	American Association for Automotive Medicine

1

AAAS ....American Association for the Advancement of Science

AABB ....American Association of Blood Banks

AACC ....American Association of Clinical Chemists

AACO ....American Association of Certified Orthoptists

AACP ....American Association of Colleges of Pharmacy

AACR ....American Association for Cancer Research

AAD ....American Academy of Dermatology

AADP ....American Academy of Denture Prosthetics

AADS ....American Association of Dental Schools

AAE ....American Association of Endodontists

AAEE ....American Academy of Environmental Engineers

AAF.............acetaminofluorene

AAGP ....American Academy of General Practice

AAHM ....American Association of the History of Medicine

AAHP ....Army artificial heart pump

AAI ....American Association of Immunologists

AAIN ....American Association of Industrial Nurses

AALAS ....American Association of Laboratory Animal Science

AAMA..........American Association of Medical Assistants

AAMC..........American Association of Medical Clinics
　　　　　　　　Association of American Medical Colleges

AAMD ....American Association on Mental Deficiency

AAME..........acetylarginine methyl ester

AAMI...........Association for the Advancement of Medical Instrumentation

AAMRL ....American Association of Medical Record Librarians

AAN ....American Academy of Neurology

AANA..........American Association of Nurse Anesthetists

AANS ....American Academy of Neurological Surgery
　　　　　　　　American Association of Neurological Surgeons

AAO ....American Association of Ophthalmology
　　　　　　　　American Association of Orthodontists

AAOG ....American Association of Obstetricians and Gynecologists

AAOO ....American Academy of Ophthalmology and Otolaryngology

AAOP ....American Academy of Oral Pathology

AAOS ....American Academy of Orthopaedic Surgeons

AAP.............air at atmospheric pressure
　　　　　　　　American Academy of Pediatrics

AAP *Continued*

American Academy of Pedodontics
American Academy of Periodontology
Association of American Physicians
AAPB ....American Association of Pathologists and Bacteriologists
AAPMR ....American Academy of Physical Medicine and Rehabilitation
AAPPP ....American Association of Planned Parenthood Physicians
AAPS...........Association of American Physicians and Surgeons
AAR ....antigen-antiglobulin reaction
AARS ....American Association of Railway Surgeons
AAS.............aortic arch syndrome
AASCU........American Association of State Colleges and Universities
AAT.............alpha-antitrypsin
AB...............abnormal
abortion
alcian blue
American Board
asbestos body
asthmatic bronchitis
axiobuccal
A/B..............acid-base ratio
ABA ....antibacterial activity
ABC ....absolute basophil count
axiobuccocervical
ABCC..........Atomic Bomb Casualty Commission
ABD ....abdomen
abdominal
ABD HYST...abdominal hysterectomy
ABDOM ....abdomen
abdominal
ABE ....acute bacterial endocarditis
ABG ....axiobuccogingival
ABHP..........American Board of Health Physics
ABL ....a-beta-lipoproteinemia
axiobuccolingual
ABLB ....alternate binaural loudness balance
ABMS..........Advisory Board for Medical Specialties

ABN ....abnormal
ABNORM.....abnormal
ABO ....absent bed occupancy
　　　　　　　blood groups (named for agglutinogens)
ABP ....arterial blood pressure
ABRET........American Board of Registration of Electroen-
　　　　　　　cephalographic Technicians
ABS FEB.....while the fever is absent (*absente febre*)
AC..............acromioclavicular
　　　　　　　acute
　　　　　　　adrenal cortex
　　　　　　　air conduction
　　　　　　　alternating current
　　　　　　　anodal closure
　　　　　　　anticoagulant
　　　　　　　anticomplementary
　　　　　　　anti-inflammatory corticoid
　　　　　　　aortic closure
　　　　　　　atriocarotid
　　　　　　　auriculocarotid
　　　　　　　axiocervical
　　　　　　　—before meals (*ante cibum*)
ACA ....adenocarcinoma
　　　　　　　American Chiropractic Association
　　　　　　　American College of Allergists
　　　　　　　American College of Anesthesiologists
ACAD..........academy
ACC ....adenoid cystic carcinoma
　　　　　　　American College of Cardiology
　　　　　　　anodal closing contraction
ACCESS ......American College of Cardiology Extended Study
　　　　　　　Services
ACCL ....anodal closure clonus
ACCP ....American College of Chest Physicians
ACD ....absolute cardiac dulness
　　　　　　　acid, citrate, dextrose
　　　　　　　anterior chest diameter
ACE ....adrenocortical extract
　　　　　　　alcohol, chloroform, ether
ACEP ....American College of Emergency Physicians

ACFO ....American College of Foot Orthopedists
ACFS...........American College of Foot Surgeons
ACG ....apexcardiogram
Ac-G ....accelerator globulin
ACH ....adrenal cortical hormone
ACh ....acetylcholine
ACHA ....American College Health Association
ACHE ....acetylcholinesterase
ACIP ....Advisory Committee on Immunization Practices
ACl..............aspiryl chloride
ACM ....albumin-calcium-magnesium
ACO ....anodal closing odor
ACOG ....American College of Obstetricians and Gynecologists
ACOS ....American College of Osteopathic Surgeons
ACP.............acid phosphatase
                acyl-carrier protein
                American College of Physicians
                anodal closing picture
                aspirin, caffein, phenacetin
ACPM..........American College of Preventive Medicine
ACR ....American College of Radiology
ACS.............American Cancer Society
                American Chemical Society
                American College of Surgeons
                anodal closing sound
                antiroticular cytotoxic serum
ACSW..........Academy of Certified Social Workers
ACT.............activated coagulation time
                anticoagulant therapy
ACTe ....anodal closure tetanus
ACTH ....adrenocorticotropic hormone
ACTP...........adrenocorticotropin polypeptide
ACVD ....acute cardiovascular disease
AD..............admitting diagnosis
                Aleutian disease
                anodal duration
                average deviation
                axiodistal
                axis deviation
                right ear (*auris dextra*)
A & D...........ascending and descending

AD DEF AN to the point of fainting (*ad defectionem animi*)
AD GRAT ACID...to an agreeable sourness (*ad gratum acid-itatem*)
AD LIB........as desired (*ad libitum*)
AD POND OM...to the weight of the whole (*ad pondus omnium*)
AD 2 VIC.....for two doses (*ad duas vices*)
ADA ....adenosine deaminase
              American Dental Association
              American Dermatological Association
              American Diabetes Association
              American Dietetic Association
              anterior descending artery
ADA# ....American Diabetes Association diet number
ADAA..........American Dental Assistants Association
ADC ....Aid to Dependent Children
              anodal duration contraction
              average daily census
              axiodistocervical
ADEM ....acute disseminated encephalomyelitis
ADG ....axiodistogingival
ADH ....alcohol dehydrogenase
              antidiuretic hormone
ADHA..........American Dental Hygienists Association
ADHIB ....to be administered (*adhibendus*)
ADI ....axiodistoincisal
ADL ....activities of daily living
ADM............administrative medicine
              administrator
              admission
              admit
ADMOV ....let there be added (*admove*)
ADN ....Associate Degree in Nursing
ADO ....axiodisto-occlusal
ADP ....adenosine diphosphate
              automatic data processing
ADPL ....average daily patient load
ADS.............antibody deficiency syndrome
              antidiuretic substance
ADT.............adenosine triphosphate
              any thing desired
ADV ....against (*adversum*)

AEC ....Atomic Energy Commission
AEG ....air encephalogram
               the patient (*aeger*)
AEP............average evoked potential
AER ....aldosterone excretion rate
               auditory evoked response
               average evoked response
AES............American Epidemiological Society
AET............absorption-equivalent thickness
               age (*aetas*)
               aged (*aetatis*)
AF ....acid-fast
               aldehyde fuchsin
               amniotic fluid
               antibody-forming
               aortic flow
               atrial fibrillation
               atrial flutter
AFB ....acid-fast bacillus
               American Foundation for the Blind
AFC............antibody-forming cells
AFCR ....American Federation for Clinical Research
AFDC ....Aid to Families of Dependent Children
AFI............amaurotic familial idiocy
AFIB ....atrial fibrillation
AFIP ....Air Force Institute of Pathology
AFL............atrial flutter
AFP............anterior faucial pillar
AFQT..........Armed Forces Qualification Test
AG.............antiglobulin
               atrial gallop
               axiogingival
A/G............albumin-globulin ratio
AGA ....American Gastroenterological Association
               American Goiter Association
               appropriate for gestational age
AGG ....agammaglobulinemia
               aggravated
AGGRED FEB...while the fever is coming on (*aggrediente febre*)
AGIT ....shake
AGIT VAS ...the vial being shaken (*agitato vase*)

AGL.............acute granulocytic leukemia
               aminoglutethimide
AGMK.........African green monkey kidney
AGN.............acute glomerulonephritis
AGS.............adrenogenital syndrome
               American Gynecological Society
AGT.............antiglobulin test
AGTT...........abnormal glucose tolerance test
AGV.............aniline gentian violet
AH...............abdominal hysterectomy
               acetohexamide
               amenorrhea and hirsutism
               aminohippurate
               antihyaluronidase
               arterial hypertension
               hypermetropic astigmatism
AHA.............acquired hemolytic anemia
               American Heart Association
               American Hospital Association
               autoimmune hemolytic anemia
AHD.............atherosclerotic heart disease
AHEA.........American Home Economics Association
AHF.............antihemophilic factor
AHG.............antihemophilic globulin
               antihuman globulin
AHH.............alpha-hydrazine analogue of histidine
               arylhydrocarbon hydroxylase
AHLE.........acute hemorrhagic leukoencephalitis
AHLS.........antihuman-lymphocyte serum
AHP.............air at high pressure
AHS.............Adult Health Study
               American Hearing Society
AHT.............augmented histamine test
AI...............accidentally incurred
               aortic incompetence
               aortic insufficiency
               apical impulse
               axioincisal
AIB.............aminoisobutyric acid
AIBCS.........American Intersociety Board of Certification of
               Sanitarians

AIC ....aminoimidazole carboxamide
AID ....Agency for International Development
                America-India Dispensary
                artificial insemination, donor
AIEP ....amount of insulin extractable from the pancreas
AIH ....artificial insemination, homologous
AIHA...........American Industrial Hygiene Association
                autoimmune hemolytic anemia
AIN ....American Institute of Nutrition
AIP...............acute intermittent porphyria
                average intravascular pressure
AIU ....absolute iodine uptake
AJ ....ankle jerk
AK................above knee
AKA ....above-knee amputation
AL................albumin
                axiolingual
ALA.............American Laryngological Association
                aminolevulinic acid
                axiolabial
ALAD ....abnormal left axis deviation
                aminolevulinic acid dehydrase
ALAG ....axiolabiogingival
ALB ....albumin
                white
ALC.............approximate lethal concentration
                axiolinguocervical
ALD ....aldolase
ALG.............antilymphocyte globulin
                axiolinguogingival
ALH ....anterior lobe hormone
                anterior lobe of the hypophysis
ALIMD ....Association of Life Insurance Medical Directors
ALK ....alkaline
ALK PHOS...alkaline phosphatase
ALL.............acute lymphoblastic leukemia
                acute lymphocytic leukemia
                allergies
ALME..........acetyl-lysine methyl ester
ALMI...........anterior lateral myocardial infarct
ALN ....anterior lymph node

ALO..............axiolinguo-occlusal
ALP..............alkaline phosphatase
　　　　　antilymphocyte plasma
ALROS ....American Laryngological, Rhinological and Oto-
　　　　　logical Society
ALS..............amyotrophic lateral sclerosis
　　　　　antilymphatic serum
　　　　　antilymphocyte serum
ALT DIEB ...every other day (*alternis diebus*)
ALT HOR....every other hour (*alternis horis*)
ALT NOC.....every other night (*alternis nocte*)
ALTEE ....acetyl-L-tyrosine ethyl ester
ALV ADST...when the bowels are constipated (*alvo adstricta*)
ALV DEJECT...alvine dejections
ALW.............arch-loop-whorl
AM..............alveolar macrophage
　　　　　ametropia
　　　　　amperemeter
　　　　　anovular menstruation
　　　　　arithmetic mean
　　　　　aviation medicine
　　　　　axiomesial
　　　　　morning
　　　　　myopic astigmatism
am...............meter-angle
AMA...........against medical advice
　　　　　American Medical Association
　　　　　Australian Medical Association
AMAERF .....American Medical Association Education and Re-
　　　　　search Foundation
AMAL..........Aero-Medical Acceleration Laboratory
AMB............ambulatory
AMC............axiomesiocervical
AMCAS........American Medical College Application Service
AMD............alpha-methyldopa
　　　　　axiomesiodistal
AMDOC ....American doctor
AMDS..........Association of Military Dental Surgeons
AME............Aviation Medical Examiners
AMEL..........Aero-Medical Equipment Laboratory
AMG............antimacrophage globulin
　　　　　axiomesiogingival

AMH............automated medical history
mixed astigmatism with myopia predominating
AMI.............acute myocardial infarction
amitriptyline
Association of Medical Illustrators
axiomesioincisal
AML............acute monocytic leukemia
acute myelocytic leukemia
AMLS..........antimouse lymphocyte serum
AMM...........agnogenic myeloid metaplasia
ammonia
AMML.........acute myelomonocytic leukemia
AMO............axiomesio-occlusal
AMOL..........acute monocytic leukemia
AMP............acid mucopolysaccharide
adenosine monophosphate
ampicillin
amputation
average mean pressure
amp.............ampere
AMPAC.......American Medical Political Action Committee
AMPS..........abnormal mucopolysacchariduria
acid mucopolysaccharides
AMRA..........American Medical Record Association
AMS............aggravated in military service
antimacrophage serum
automated multiphasic screening
AMSUS........Association of Military Surgeons of the United
States
AMT............alpha-methyltyrosine
amethopterin
amount
AMWA.........American Medical Women's Association
American Medical Writers' Association
AMY............amylase
AN...............anterior
ANA............acetylneuraminic acid
American Neurological Association
American Nurses' Association
antinuclear antibodies
aspartyl naphthylamide

ANAL .... analysis
               analyst
ANAT .... anatomical
               anatomy
ANC .... Army Nurse Corps
ANCC .... anodal closure contraction
ANES .... anesthesia
               anesthesiology
ANESTH ...... anesthesia
               anesthesiology
ANF .... alpha-naphthoflavone
               antinuclear factor
ANG .... angiogram
ANHA .... American Nursing Home Association
ANK .... ankle
ANOC .... anodal opening contraction
ANOV .... analysis of variance
ANS .... antineutrophilic serum
               arteriolonephrosclerosis
               autonomic nervous system
ANT .... anterior
ANTE .... before
ANTR .... apparent net transfer rate
ANTU .... alpha-naphthylthiourea
AO .... anodal opening
               anterior oblique
               aorta
               aortic opening
               axio-occlusal
               opening of the atrioventricular valves
AOA .... American Orthopedic Association
               American Osteopathic Association
AOB .... alcohol on breath
AOC .... anodal opening contraction
AOCL .... anodal opening clonus
AOD .... arterial occlusive disease
AOM .... Master of Obstetric Art
AOO .... anodal opening odor
AOP .... anodal opening picture
AOS .... American Ophthalmological Society
               American Otological Society

AOS *Continued*
    anodal opening sound
AOTA ....American Occupational Therapy Association
AOTe ....anodal opening tetanus
AP...............Academy of Periodontology
    acid phosphatase
    action potential
    acute proliferative
    alkaline phosphatase
    aminopeptidase
    angina pectoris
    antepartum
    anterior pituitary
    anteroposterior
    appendix
    arterial pressure
    association period
    axiopulpal
A&P ....anterior and posterior
    auscultation and palpation
APA..............aldosterone-producing adenoma
    American Pharmaceutical Association
    American Physiotherapy Association
    American Podiatry Association
    American Psychiatric Association
    American Psychoanalytic Association
    American Psychological Association
    aminopenicillanic acid
    antipernicious anemia factor
APB ....atrial premature beat
    auricular premature beat
APC..............acetylsalicylic acid, phenacetin, caffeine
    adenoidal-pharyngeal-conjunctival
    aspirin, phenacetin, caffeine
    atrial premature contraction
APCA ....Air Pollution Control Association
APC-C ....aspirin, phenacetin, caffeine; with codeine
APD ....action potential duration
APE..............adapted physical educator
    aminophylline, phenobarbital, ephedrine
    anterior pituitary extract

APF ....animal protein factor
APGL ....alkaline phosphatase activity of the granular leuko-
                cytes
APH ....antepartum hemorrhage
APHA ....American Protestant Hospital Association
                American Public Health Association
APHP ....antipseudomonas human plasma
APIM...........Association   Professionelle   Internationale   des
                Médecins
APL............accelerated painless labor
                anterior pituitary-like
APM ....Academy of Physical Medicine
APN ....average peak noise
APP.............alum-precipitated pyridine
                appendix
APPY ....appendectomy
APR............amebic prevalence rate
APS ....American Proctologic Society
APT.............alum-precipitated toxoid
APTA...........American Physical Therapy Association
APTT ....activated partial thromboplastin time
AQ..............achievement quotient
                water (*aqua*)
AQ BULL.....boiling water (*aqua bulliens*)
AQ DEST....distilled water (*aqua destillata*)
AQ FERV.....hot water (*aqua fervens*)
AQ FRIG......cold water (*aqua frigida*)
AQ PUR.......pure water (*aqua pura*)
AQ TEP ....tepid water (*aqua tepida*)
AQS............additional qualifying symptoms
AR..............alarm reaction
                aortic regurgitation
                Argyll Robertson (pupil)
                artificial respiration
                at risk
ARA ....American Rheumatism Association
ARC ....American Red Cross
                anomalous retinal correspondence
                average response computer
ARD ....acute respiratory disease
                anorectal dressing

ARF.............acute respiratory failure
American Rehabilitation Foundation
ARG ....silver
ARL.............average remaining lifetime
ARM............artificial rupture of the membranes
ARMH ....Academy of Religion and Mental Health
ARP.............at risk period
ARPA ....Advanced Research Projects Agency
ARRT ....American Registry of Radiologic Technologists
ARS.............Agricultural Research Service
American Rhinologic Society
antirabies serum
ART.............Accredited Record Technician
artery
AS ....acetylstrophanthidin
Adams-Stokes (disease)
androsterone sulfate
antistreptolysin
aortic stenosis
arteriosclerosis
left ear (*auris sinistra*)
ASA.............acetylsalicylic acid
Acoustical Society of America
Adams-Stokes attack
American Society of Anesthesiologists
American Standards Association
arylsulfatase-A
ASAIO ....American Society for Artificial Internal Organs
ASC.............American Society of Cytology
ASCC ....American Society for the Control of Cancer
ASCI ....American Society for Clinical Investigation
ASCP...........American Society of Clinical Pathologists
ASCPC ....American Society of Clinical Pharmacology and
Chemotherapy
ASCVD ....arteriosclerotic cardiovascular disease
atherosclerotic cardiovascular disease
ASD.............aldosterone secretion defect
atrial septal defect
ASDR ....American Society of Dental Radiographers
ASEP...........American Society for Experimental Pathology
ASF.............aniline, formaldehyde, and sulfur

ASG..............American Society for Genetics
ASGE ....American Society of Gastrointestinal Endoscopy
ASH..............Action on Smoking and Health
                hypermetropic astigmatism
ASHA ....American Social Health Association
                American Speech and Hearing Association
ASHD ....arteriosclerotic heart disease
ASHP ....American Society of Hospital Pharmacists
ASIM...........American Society of Internal Medicine
ASIS............anterior superior iliac spine
ASK.............antistreptokinase
ASL..............American Sign Language
                antistreptolysin
ASLO...........antistreptolysin-O
ASM ....myopic astigmatism
ASMI...........anteroseptal myocardial infarct
ASMT ....American Society of Medical Technologists
ASN.............alkali-soluble nitrogen
ASO..............American Society of Orthodontists
                antistreptolysin-O
                arteriosclerosis obliterans
ASP..............American Society of Parasitologists
                area systolic pressure
ASR.............aldosterone secretion rate
                aldosterone secretory rate
ASS ....anterior superior spine
ASST...........assistant
AST ....astigmatism
ASTH...........asthenopia
ASTO...........antistreptolysin-O
ASTR...........American Society of Therapeutic Radiologists
ASV.............antisnake venom
AT ....antitrypsin
AT WT ....atomic weight
ATA.............anti-Toxoplasma antibodies
                atmosphere absolute
                aurintricarboxylic acid
ATB.............at the time of the bombing
ATCC ....American Type Culture Collections
ATD.............Aid to Totally Disabled
                asphyxiating thoracic dystrophy

ATE ....adipose tissue extract
ATEE ....acetyltyrosine ethyl ester
ATG ....antithyroglobulin
ATN ....acute tubular necrosis
ATP ....adenosine triphosphate
ATPS ....ambient temperature and pressure, saturated with water vapor
ATR ....Achilles tendon reflex
ATR FIB ......atrial fibrillation
ATS ....American Therapeutic Society
American Thoracic Society
antitetanic serum
antithymocyte serum
anxiety tension state
arteriosclerosis
ATT ....aspirin tolerance time
attending
AU ....Angstrom unit
antitoxin unit
arbitrary units
Australia (antigen)
azauridine
both ears (*aures unitas*)
AUA ....American Urological Association
AUHAA ....Australia-hepatitis associated antigen
AUL ....acute undifferentiated leukemia
AUPHA ....Association of University Programs in Hospital Administration
AUPO ....Association of University Professors of Ophthalmology
AUR FIB .....auricular fibrillation
AUSC ....auscultation
AV ....arteriovenous
atrioventricular
AV/AF ....anteverted, anteflexed
AVCS ....atrioventricular conduction system
AVF ....arteriovenous fistula
AVH ....acute viral hepatitis
AVI ....air velocity index
AVMA ....American Veterinary Medical Association
AVN ....atrioventricular node

AVR ....aortic valve replacement
AVRP ....atrioventricular refractory period
AVT............Allen vision test
AW ....anterior wall
A&W............alive and well
AWI.............anterior wall infarction
AWMI..........anterior wall myocardial infarction
AX...............axis
AZG............azaguanine
AZO-...........(indicates presence of the group) -N:N-
AZT ....Aschheim-Zondek test
AZUR ....azauridine

B

B ....bacillus
base
bath (*balneum*)
Baumé's scale
behavior
Benoist's scale
bicuspid
born
Brucella
buccal
symbol of gauss
B4 ....before
BA...............bacterial agglutination
betamethasone acetate
blocking antibody
bone age
bovine albumin
brachial artery
bronchial asthma
buccoaxial
BAC ....blood alcohol concentration
buccoaxiocervical
BACT ....bacterium
BAEE ....benzoyl arginine ethyl ester
benzylarginine ethyl ester
BAG ....buccoaxiogingival
BAIB...........beta-aminoisobutyric acid
BAL ....bath
British Anti-Lewisite
BALS ....balsam
BAME ....benzoylarginine methyl ester
BAO ....basal acid output
BAP ....blood agar plate
BAS.............Battalion Aid Station
BASH ....body acceleration given synchronously with the
heartbeat
BB ....blood bank
blood buffer base
blue bloaters (emphysema)

BB *Continued*
- both bones
- breakthrough bleeding
- breast biopsy
- buffer base

BBB ....blood-brain barrier
- bundle branch block

BBT ....basal body temperature

BC......ˌ........bactericidal concentration
- battle casualty
- Blue Cross
- bone conduction
- buccocervical

BCA ....Blue Cross Association

BCB ....brilliant cresyl blue

BCE ....basal cell epithelioma

BCG ....bacille Calmette Guérin
- ballistocardiogram
- bicolor guaiac (test)

BCNU..........bischloroethyl-nitrosourea
- bischloronitrosourea

BCR ....Beryllium Case Registry

BCW............biological and chemical warfare

BD ....base deficit
- base of prism down
- bile duct
- buccodistal
- twice a day (*bis die*)

BDA ....British Dental Association

BDE ....bile duct exploration

BDI ....Beck Depression Inventory

BDS ....Bachelor of Dental Surgery

BDSc ....Bachelor of Dental Science

BE...............bacterial endocarditis
- barium enema
- base excess
- bovine enteritis

BEI ....butanol-extractable iodine

BEV ....billion electron volts

BF...............blood flow
- bouillon filtrate (tuberculin)

B/F..............bound-free ratio
BFC ....benign febrile convulsion
BFP..............biologic false-positive
BFR ....biologic false-positive reactor
              blood flow rate
              bone formation rate
BFT..............bentonite flocculation test
BG...............blood glucose
              bone graft
              buccogingival
BGH ....bovine growth hormone
BGP ....beta-glycerophosphatase
BGSA ....blood granulocyte-specific activity
BGTT...........borderline glucose tolerance test
BH ....benzalkonium and heparin
BHA ....butylated hydroxyanisole
BHC ....benzene hexachloride
BHI ....brain-heart infusion
BHS ....beta-hemolytic streptococcus
BHT ....butylated hydroxytoluene
BH/VH.........body hematocrit-venous hematocrit ratio
BI................bacteriological index
              base of prism in
              burn index
BIB.............drink (*bibe*)
BID.............twice a day (*bis in die*)
BIDLB ....block in the postero-inferior division of the left
                  branch
BIH ....benign intracranial hypertension
BIL ....bilateral
              bilirubin
BILAT.........bilateral
BIN ....twice a night (*bis in nocte*)
BIP ....bismuth iodoform paraffin
BIS..............twice
BJ ....Bence Jones
BJP ....Bence Jones protein
BK ....below knee
BKA ....below-knee amputation
BKFST ....breakfast

BL...............baseline
Bessey-Lowry (units)
bleeding
blood loss
buccolingual
Burkitt's lymphoma
BL PR ....blood pressure
BLB ....Boothby, Lovelace, Bulbulian (mask)
BLG ....beta-lactoglobulin
BLN ....bronchial lymph nodes
BLOT ....British Library of Tape Recordings
BLT............blood-clot lysis time
BLU ....Bessey-Lowry units
BM ....Bachelor of Medicine
basement membrane
body mass
bone marrow
bowel movement
buccomesial
sea-water bath (*balneum maris*)
BMA............British Medical Association
BMK............birth mark
BMR............basal metabolic rate
BMS ....Bachelor of Medical Science
BN ....brachial neuritis
BNA ....Basle Nomina Anatomica
BNDD ....Bureau of Narcotics and Dangerous Drugs
BNO ....bladder-neck obstruction
BNPA..........binasal pharyngeal airway
BO...............base of prism out
bowel obstruction
bucco-occlusal
B&O ....belladonna and opium
BOL ....pill (*bolus*)
BOM............bilateral otitis media
BP...............Bachelor of Pharmacy
back pressure
bathroom privileges
behavior pattern
benzopyrene
birthplace

BP *Continued*

       blood pressure
       boiling point
       British Pharmacopeia
       bronchopleural
       buccopulpal

BPC ....British Pharmaceutical Codex
BPH ....benign prostatic hypertrophy
BPh ....British Pharmacopeia
BPL.............beta-propiolactone
BPO ....benzylpenicilloyl
BPRS ....brief psychiatric rating scale
       brief psychiatric reacting scale
BR...............bathroom
       bed rest
       bilirubin
       British Revision of Basle Nomina Anatomica
       Brucella
BRBC..........bovine red blood cells
BRH ....Bureau of Radiological Health
BRKF..........breakfast
BRKT ....breakfast
BRM............biuret reactive material
BRP ....bathroom privileges
       bilirubin production
BRTH ....breath
BS ....Bachelor of Surgery
       Beauty Shop (hospital)
       blood sugar
       Blue Shield
       bowel sounds
       breaking strength
       breath sounds
BSA.............bismuth-sulphite agar
       body surface area
       bovine serum albumin
BSB ....body surface burned
BSDLB........block in the anterosuperior division of the left
               branch
BSF.............back scatter factor
BSI..............bound serum iron

BSO..............bilateral salpingo-oophorectomy
BSP..............Bromsulphalein
BSR..............basal skin resistance
BSS..............balanced salt solution
                        black silk suture
                        buffered saline solution
BSU............British Standard Units
BT................bladder tumor
                        brain tumor
BTB............breakthrough bleeding
BThU...........British Thermal Unit
BTPS...........body temperature, ambient pressure, saturated
                        with water
BTR.............Bezold-type reflex
BTU............British Thermal Unit
BU..............base of prism up
                        Bodansky units
                        burn unit
BUDR..........bromodeoxyuracil
                        bromodeoxyuridine
BULL..........let it boil (*bulliat*)
BUN............blood urea nitrogen
BUPA..........British United Provident Association
BUT............butter
BV...............biologic value
                        blood vessel
                        blood volume
                        bronchovesicular
                        vapor bath
BVH............biventricular hypertrophy
BVI.............blood vessel invasion
BVSc...........Bachelor of Veterinary Science
BVV............bovine vaginitis virus
BW..............biological warfare
                        birth weight
                        body water
                        body weight
BX...............biopsy

C

C ....calculus
calorie (large)
canine
carbohydrate
cathode
Caucasian
Celsius
centigrade
certified
cervical
chest
clearance rate
clonus
Clostridium
closure
color sense
compound
contracture
correct
Cryptococcus
cup
cylinder
gallon
hundred
velocity of light
C_{alb} ....albumin clearance
C_{am} ....amylase clearance
C_{cr} ....creatinine clearance
C_{in} ....insulin clearance
C_{PAH} ....para-aminohippurate clearance
C_u ....urea clearance
C' ....complement
c ....calorie (small)
curie
with (*cum*)
c' ....coefficient of partage
CA ....cancer
carcinoma
cardiac arrest

CA *Continued*

                    cathode
                    cervicoaxial
                    chronological age
                    cold agglutinin
                    common antigen
                    coronary artery
                    corpora amylacea
                    croup associated (virus)
ca ....about (*circa*)
CACC ....cathodal closure contraction
CAD ....coronary artery disease
CADTe.........cathodal duration tetanus
CAG ....chronic atrophic gastritis
CAH ....chronic active hepatitis
                    congenital adrenal hyperplasia
CAHD..........coronary atherosclerotic heart disease
CAI ....computer-assisted instruction
CAL.............computer-assisted learning
Cal ....large calorie
cal ....small calorie
CALEF ....warmed (*calefactus*)
CAM............chorioallantoic membrane
                    contralateral axillary metastasis
CAMP..........computer-assisted menu planning
                    cyclic adenosine monophosphate
CAO ....chronic airway obstruction
CAP.............capsule
                    cellulose acetate phthalate
                    chloramphenicol
                    College of American Pathologists
                    cystine aminopeptidase
                    let him take (*capiat*)
CARD..........cardiology
CARDIOL ...cardiology
CARF ....Commission on Accreditation of Rehabilitation
                    Facilities
CAS..............Cancer Attitude Survey
CAT.............Children's Apperception Test
                    Computer of Average Transients

CATH ....cathartic
              catheter
              catheterize
CAV ....congenital absence of vagina
              congenital adrenal virilism
CB...............Bachelor of Surgery
              chronic bronchitis
CBA ....chronic bronchitis with asthma
CBC ....complete blood count
CBD ....common bile duct
CBE ....Council of Biology Editors
CBF ....cerebral blood flow
              coronary blood flow
CBG ....corticosteroid-binding globulin
              cortisol-binding globulin
CBOC..........completion bed occupancy care
CBS.............chronic brain syndrome
CBV ....central blood volume
              circulating blood volume
              corrected blood volume
CBW............chemical and biological warfare
CC...............cardiac cycle
              chief complaint
              clinical course
              commission certified   — with
              compound cathartic
              cord compression
              costochondral
              creatinine clearance
cc ....cubic centimeter
CCA ....chick-cell agglutination
              chimpanzee coryza agent
              common carotid artery
CCAT ....conglutinating complement absorption test
CCC ....cathodal closing contraction
              chronic calculous cholecystitis
              Commission on Clinical Chemistry
              consecutive case conference
CCCL ....cathodal closure clonus
CCF.............cephalin-cholesterol flocculation

CCF *Continued*
               compound comminuted fracture
               congestive cardiac failure
CCK ....cholecystokinin
CCK-PZ ....cholecystokinin pancreozymin
CCN ....coronary care nursing
CCNSC ....Cancer Chemotherapy National Service Center
CCP.............ciliocytophthoria
CCS.............casualty clearing station
CCT.............composite cyclic therapy
CCTe ....cathodal closure tetanus
CCTP...........Coronary Care Training Project
CCU ....Cherry-Crandall units
               community care unit
               coronary care unit
CCW............counterclockwise
CD...............cadaver donor
               cardiac disease
               cardiac dulness
               cardiovascular disease
               caudal
               common duct
               conjugata diagonalis
               consanguineous donor
               curative dose
               cystic duct
C/D..............cigarettes per day
C&D ....cystoscopy and dilatation
CD$_{50}$............median curative dose
CDC ....calculated day of confinement
               chenodeoxycholate
               Communicable Disease Center
CDD ....certificate of disability for discharge
CDE ....canine distemper encephalitis
               chlordiazepoxide
               common duct exploration
CDH ....ceramide dihexoside
               congenital dislocation of the hip
CDL ....chlorodeoxylincomycin
CDP ....coronary drug project
CDSS...........clinical decision support system

CE...............California encephalitis
cardiac enlargement
chick embryo
cholesterol esters
contractile element
CEA ....carcino-embryonic antigen
crystalline egg albumin
CEEV ....Central European encephalitis virus
CEF.............chick embryo fibroblast
CEL.............Celsius
CENT ....Centigrade
cent ....centimeter
centi- ....hundred
CEPH FLOC...cephalin flocculation
CERT ....certified
CES.............central excitatory state
CF ....carbolfuchsin
cardiac failure
carrier-free
chemotactic factor
chest and left leg
Chiari-Frommel syndrome
Christmas factor
citrovorum factor
compare
complement fixation
complement-fixing
contractile force
count fingers
counting finger
cystic fibrosis
CFA.............complement-fixing antibody
complete Freund adjuvant
CFF.............critical flicker fusion test
critical fusion frequency
CFP.............chronic false-positive
cystic fibrosis of the pancreas
CFSTI..........Clearinghouse for Federal Scientific and Technical
Information
CFT.............clinical full-time
complement fixation test

CFU ....colony-forming units
color-forming units
CFWM ....cancer-free white mouse
CG...............cardio-green
chorionic gonadotropin
chronic glomerulonephritis
colloidal gold
phosgene
cg ....centigram
CGD ....chronic granulomatous disease
CGI ....clinical global impression
CGL.............chronic granulocytic leukemia
cgm ....centigram
CGN ....chronic glomerulonephritis
CG/OQ ....cerebral glucose oxygen quotient
CGP.............choline glycerophosphatide
chorionic growth hormone prolactin
circulating granulocyte pool
CGS.............centimeter-gram-second
CGTT...........cortisone glucose tolerance test
CH...............cholesterol
Community Health
crown-heel (length of fetus)
wheelchair
CHA ....congenital hypoplastic anemia
cyclohexylamine
CHAMPUS...Civilian Health and Medical Program of the Uni-
formed Services
CHART........paper (*charta*)
CHB ....complete heart block
CHD ....congenital heart disease
coronary heart disease
CHE ....cholinesterase
CHF ....congestive heart failure
CHH ....cartilage-hair hypoplasia
CHL ....chloramphenicol
ChM ....Master of Surgery
CHO ....carbohydrate
CHOL ....cholesterol
CHP ....child psychiatry
comprehensive health planning

CHR ....Chromobacterium
chronic
CHS............Chediak-Higashi syndrome
CHW............Community Health Week
CI................cardiac index
cardiac insufficiency
cerebral infarction
chemotherapeutic index
clinical investigator
colloidal iron
color index
coronary insufficiency
crystalline insulin
CIB ....food (*cibus*)
CICU ....cardiology intensive care unit
coronary intensive care unit
CID ....cytomegalic inclusion disease
CIDS ....cellular immunity deficiency syndrome
CIEBM ....Committee on the Interplay of Engineering with
Biology and Medicine
CIN ....cervical intra-epithelial neoplasia
CIRC ....circulation
CIS..............carcinoma in situ
central inhibitory state
CK.....,........check
creatine kinase
CL...............chest and left arm
Clostridium
cl.................centiliter
CLA............Certified Laboratory Assistant
CLAS...........congenital localized absence of skin
CLBBB ....complete left bundle branch block
CLD ....chronic liver disease
chronic lung disease
CLIN ....clinic
clinical
CLL.............chronic lymphatic leukemia
chronic lymphocytic leukemia
CLML ....Current List of Medical Literature
CLO.............cod liver oil
CLSL...........chronic lymphosarcoma (cell) leukemia

CLT ....clot-lysis time
CM ....capreomycin
                chloroquine-mepacrine
                cochlear microphonic
                complications
                costal margin
                cow's milk
                Master in Surgery
                tomorrow morning (*cras mane*)
cm ....centimeter
cm^3 ....cubic centimeter
CMA ....Canadian Medical Association
CMB ....carbolic methylene blue
CMC ....carboxymethyl cellulose
                critical micellar concentration
CME ....Continuing Medical Education
CMF ....chondromyxoid fibroma
CMGN ....chronic membranous glomerulonephritis
CMI ....carbohydrate metabolism index
                cellular-mediated immune (response)
CMID ....cytomegalic inclusion disease
c/min ....cycles per minute
CML ....chronic myelocytic leukemia
                chronic myelogenous leukemia
CMM ....cutaneous malignant melanoma
cmm.............cubic millimeter
CMN.............cystic medial necrosis
CMN-AA ......cystic medial necrosis of the ascending aorta
CMO ....cardiac minute output
                card made out
                Chief Medical Officer
CMP ....cytidine monophosphate
CMR ....cerebral metabolic rate
                Certified Medical Representative
                crude mortality ratio
CMRG..........cerebral metabolic rate of glucose
CMRO..........cerebral metabolic rate of oxygen
CMS ....Clyde Mood Scale
                to be taken tomorrow morning (*cras mane sumendus*)
CMT ....Current Medical Terminology
CMU............chlorophenyldimethylurea

CMV ....cytomegalovirus
CN...............clinical nursing
cyanogen
tomorrow night (*cras nocte*)
CNA ....Canadian Nurses' Association
CNC ....Clinical Nursing Conference
CNE ....chronic nervous exhaustion
CNH ....community nursing home
CNHD..........congenital nonspherocytic hemolytic disease
CNHI...........Committee for National Health Insurance
CNL ....cardiolipin natural lecithin
CNM............Certified Nurse-Midwife
CNS.............central nervous system
to be taken tomorrow night (*cras nocte sumendus*)
CNV ....conative negative variation
contingent negative variation
CO...............carbon monoxide
cardiac output
castor oil
cervicoaxial
coenzyme
corneal opacity
compound
C/O..............complains of
complaints
COA ....coenzyme A
COAG ....coagulation
COC ....cathodal opening clonus
coccygeal
combination-type oral contraceptive
COCHL........spoonful (*cochleare*)
COCHL AMP...heaping spoonful (*cochleare amplum*)
COCHL MAG...tablespoonful (*cochleare magnum*)
COCHL MED...dessertspoonful (*cochleare medium*)
COCHL PARV...teaspoonful (*cochleare parvum*)
COCL ....cathodal opening clonus
COCT ....boiling (*coctio*)
COD ....cause of death
COGTT.........cortisone-primed oral glucose tolerance test
COHB..........carboxyhemoglobin
COL.............strain (*cola*)

COLAT ....strained (*colatus*)
COLD ....chronic obstructive lung disease
COLL ....eyewash (*collyrium*)
COLLUT......mouth wash (*collutorium*)
COLLYR......eyewash
COMP..........complaint
complication
compound
COMT..........catechol-*O*-methyl transferase
CONC..........concentration
CONCIS.......cut (*concisus*)
cong.............gallon
CONT ....continue
continuously
CONT REM...let the medicine be continued (*continuetur remedium*)
CONV ....conventional (rat)
COP..............colloid osmotic pressure
COPD ....chronic obstructive pulmonary disease
COPE ....Committee on Political Education
COQ ....boil (*coque*)
COQ IN S A...boil in sufficient water (*coque in sufficiente aqua*)
COQ S A ......boil properly (*coque secundum artem*)
COR ....heart
CORA ....conditioned orientation reflex audiometry
CORT ....bark
cortex
COT..............critical off-time
COTH ....Council of Teaching Hospitals
CP ....candle power
cerebral palsy
chemically pure
chloropurine
chloroquine and primaquine
chronic pyelonephritis
closing pressure
cochlear potential
combination product
combining power
coproporphyrin
creatine phosphate

C/P ....cholesterol-phospholipid ratio
C&P ....compensation and pension
CPA.............cerebellar pontine angle
                 chlorophenylalanine
CPB ....cardiopulmonary bypass
CPC.............cetylpyridinium chloride
                 chronic passive congestion
                 clinicopathologic conference
CPD ....cephalopelvic disproportion
                 citrate-phosphate-dextrose
                 compound
CPE.............chronic pulmonary emphysema
                 compensation, pension, and education
                 cytopathic effect
CPEHS ....Consumer Protection and Environmental Health
                 Service
CPH ....Certificate in Public Health
CPHA ....Committee on Professional and Hospital Activities
CPI..............constitutional psychopathic inferiority
                 Consumer Price Index
                 coronary prognostic index
CPIB ....chlorophenoxyisobutyrate
CPK ....creatine phosphokinase
cpm ....counts per minute
CPN ....chronic pyelonephritis
CPP.............cyclopentenophenanthrene
CPPB ....continuous positive-pressure breathing
CPPD ....calcium pyrophosphate dihydrate
CPR.............cerebral-cortex perfusion rate
                 cortisol production rate
CPS ....clinical performance score
                 cumulative probability of success
cps...............cycles per second
CPT ....chest physiotherapy
CPZ.............chlorpromazine
CQ..............chloroquine-quinine
                 circadian quotient
CQUCC........Commission on Quantities and Units in Clinical
                 Chemistry
CR...............calculus removed
                 chest and right arm

CR *Continued*
                 clinical research
                 colon resection
                 complete remission
                 conditioned reflex
                 crown-rump (length of fetus)
CRA ....central retinal artery
CRBBB ....complete right bundle branch block
CRD ....chronic renal disease
                 complete reaction of degeneration
CREAT ....creatinine
CRF.............chronic renal failure
                 corticotropin-releasing factor
CRI ....concentrated rust-inhibitor
CRM ....cross-reacting material
CRNA ....Certified Registered Nurse Anesthetist
CROS ....contralateral routing of signal
CRP.............C-reactive protein
CRS.............colon-rectal surgery
CRST...........calcinosis cutis, Raynaud's phenomenon, sclero-
                 dactyly, and telangiectasis
CRT.............cathode ray tube
CRU ....clinical research unit
CRV ....central retinal vein
CRYS ....crystal
CS...............Central Service
                 Central Supply
                 cesarean section
                 chondroitin sulfate
                 conditioned stimulus
                 conscious
                 coronary sinus
                 corticosteroid
                 current strength
                 cycloserine
C&S.............culture and sensitivity
CSA.............canavaninosuccinic acid
                 chondroitin sulfate-A
CSF ....cerebrospinal fluid
                 colony-stimulating factor

CSH..............chronic subdural hematoma
cortical stromal hyperplasia
CSL..............cardiolipin synthetic lecithin
CSM ....cerebrospinal meningitis
corn-soy milk
CSN..............carotid sinus nerve
CSR..............Central Supply Room
Cheyne-Stokes respiration
cortisol secretion rate
CSS ....carotid sinus stimulation
Central Sterile Supply
CST..............convulsive shock therapy
CSW ....Certified Social Worker
CT ....cardiothoracic (ratio)
carotid tracing
carpal tunnel
cerebral thrombosis
chlorothiazide
circulation time
classic technique
clotting time
coagulation time
collecting tubule
connective tissue
contraction time
Coombs' test
coronary thrombosis
corrected transposition
Corrective Therapist
corrective therapy
crest time
cytotechnologist
CTA..............Committee on Thrombolytic Agents (units)
cytotoxic assay
CTAB ....cetyltrimethylammonium bromide
CTC..............chlortetracycline
CTD..............carpal tunnel decompression
congenital thymic dysplasia
Corrective Therapy Department
CTFE...........chlorotrifluoroethylene
CTH..............ceramide trihexoside

CTR..............cardiothoracic ratio
CTZ ....chlorothiazide
CU...............color unit
                convalescent unit
cu cm...........cubic centimeter
cu mm..........cubic millimeter
CUC ....chronic ulcerative colitis
CUG ....cystourethrogram
CUJ ....of which (*cujus*)
CUJ LIB ......of any you desire (*cujus libet*)
CV ....cardiovascular
                cell volume
                central venous
                cerebrovascular
                coefficient of variation
                color vision
                conjugate diameter of pelvic inlet
                conversational voice
                corpuscular volume
                cresyl violet
                tomorrow evening (*cras vespere*)
CVA ....cardiovascular accident
                cerebrovascular accident
                costovertebral angle
CVD ....cardiovascular disease
                color vision deviant
                color vision deviate
                curved
CVH ....combined ventricular hypertrophy
CVO ....conjugate diameter of pelvic inlet
CVP.............cell volume profile
                central venous pressure
CVR ....cardiovascular-renal
                cerebrovascular resistance
CVS.............cardiovascular surgery
                cardiovascular system
                clean-voided specimen
CW ....cardiac work
                casework

CW *Continued*
        chemical warfare
        chest wall
        children's ward
        clockwise
        continuous wave
CWDF ....cell wall-deficient bacterial forms
CWI.............cardiac work index
CWP...........childbirth without pain
cwt ....hundredweight
CX...............cervix
        chest x-ray
        convex
CY...............copy
        cyanogen
CYCLO........cyclophosphamide
        cyclopropane
CYL.............cylinder

D

D ....daughter
- day
  dead
  deciduous
  density
  dermatology
  deuterium
  deuteron
  dextro
  died
  diopter
  diplomate
  distal
  divorced
  dorsal
  dose
  duration
  give (*da*)
  right (*dexter*)
  vitamin D unit
D_{CO} ....diffusing capacity for carbon monoxide
D_L ....diffusing capacity of the lung
D IN P AEQ...divide in equal parts (*divide in partes aequales*)
D TIME ....dream time
DA............degenerative arthritis
  dental assistant
  direct agglutination
  disaggregated
  dopamine
  ductus arteriosus
  give
DAB ....dimethylaminoazobenzene
DACA..........Drug Abuse Control Amendments
DAH ....disordered action of the heart
DALA ....delta-aminolevulinic acid
DAM............degraded amyloid
  diacetyl monoxime
DAO ....diamine oxidase

DAP ....dihydroxyacetone phosphate
              direct agglutination pregnancy (test)
DAPT ....Daptazole
              direct agglutination pregnancy test
DAT.............differential agglutination titer
              diphtheria antitoxin
DB ....date of birth
              dextran blue
              disability
              distobuccal
db................decibel
DBA ....dibenzanthracene
DBC ....dye binding capacity
DBCL..........dilute blood clot lysis (method)
DBI ....development-at-birth index
DBM............dibromomannitol
DBO ....distobucco-occlusal
DBP ....diastolic blood pressure
              distobuccopulpal
DBS ....Division of Biological Standards
DC...............daily census
              Dental Corps
              deoxycholate
              diagnostic code
              dilation and curettement
              diphenylarsine cyanide
              direct current
              discontinue
              distocervical
              Doctor of Chiropractic
D&C ....dilation and curettement
DCA ....deoxycholate-citrate agar
              desoxycorticosterone acetate
DCC ....double concave
DCF ....direct centrifugal flotation
DCG ....disodium cromoglycate
DCH ....Diploma in Child Health
DCHFB ....dichlorohexafluorobutane
DCI ....dichloroisoproterenol
DCT.............direct Coombs' test

DCTMA ....desoxycorticosterone trimethylacetate
DCTPA ....desoxycorticosterone triphenylacetate
DCX ....double convex
DD ....died of the disease
                differential diagnosis
                disk diameter
                let it be given to (*detur ad*)
DDC ....diethyldithiocarbamic acid
DDD............dichlorodiphenyldichloroethane
DDDIC ....Department of Defense Disease and Injury Code
DDH............Division of Dental Health
DDS ....diaminodiphenylsulfone
                Doctor of Dental Surgery
                dystrophy-dystocia syndrome
DDSc ....Doctor of Dental Science
DDT ....dichlorodiphenyltrichloroethane
DE...............dream elements
                duration of ejection
D&E ....dilation and evacuation
DE D IN D...from day to day (*de die in diem*)
DEA ....dehydroepiandrosterone
DEAE..........diethylaminoethanol
                diethylaminoethyl
DEAE-D ......diethylaminoethyl dextran
DEB SPIS ...of the proper consistency (*debita spissitudo*)
DEBA..........diethylbarbituric acid
DEC ....deceased
                deciduous
                decrease
                pour off (*decanta*)
deca-............ten
deci- ....a tenth
DECOCT......decoction
DECR..........decrease
DECUB ....lying down (*decubitus*)
DEG ....degeneration
                degree
DEGLUT......let it be swallowed (*deglutiatur*)
DEHS ....Division of Emergency Health Services
deka- ....ten
DEL ....delivery

DEM............Demerol (meperidine)
DEP ....dependents
DER ....reaction of degeneration
DERM ....dermatology
DES.............Doctors' Emergency Service
DEST...........distilled
DET.............diethyltryptamine
           give (*detur*)
DEV ....duck embryo vaccine
DF...............decapacitation factor
           degree of freedom
           desferrioxamine
           diabetic father
           discriminant function
           disseminated foci
DFDT ....difluorodiphenyltrichloroethane
DFO ....deferoxamine
DFP.............diisopropylfluorophosphate
DFU ....dead fetus in utero
           dideoxyfluorouridine
DG...............deoxyglucose
           diagnosis
           diastolic gallop
           diglyceride
           distogingival
dg...............decigram
dgm ....decigram
DH ....delayed hypersensitivity
DHA ....dehydroepiandrosterone
           dihydroxyacetone
DHAP..........dihydroxyacetone phosphate
DHAS ....dehydroepiandrosterone sulfate
DHE ....dihydroergotamine
DHEA..........dehydroepiandrosterone
DHEAS........dehydroepiandrosterone sulfate
DHEW ....Department of Health, Education, and Welfare
DHFR..........dihydrofolate reductase
DHg.............Doctor of Hygiene
DHIA...........dehydroisoandrosterone
DHN............Department of Hospital Nursing
DHT ....dihydrotachysterol

DHy.............Doctor of Hygiene
DI................diabetes insipidus
DIAG...........diagnosis
DIC ....diffuse intravascular coagulation
                disseminated intravascular coagulation
DID ....dead of intercurrent disease
DIEB ALT ...on alternate days (*diebus alternis*)
DIEB TERT...every third day (*diebus tertiis*)
DIFF ....differential
DIG ....let it be digested (*digeratur*)
DIL ....dilute
DILD...........diffuse infiltrative lung disease
DILUC.........at daybreak (*diluculo*)
DILUT.........dilute
DIM.............divalent ion metabolism
                one-half (*dimidius*)
DIME ....Division of International Medical Education
DIP ....desquamative interstitial pneumonia
                diisopropyl phosphate
                distal interphalangeal
DIPJ............distal interphalangeal joint
DIR PROP ...with proper direction
DIS..............disease
DISC ....discontinue
DISP ....dispensatory
                dispense
DIST............distill
DIT..............diiodotyrosine
DIV ....divide
DJD.............degenerative joint disease
DK ..:...........decay
                diseased kidney
                dog kidney
DL...............difference limen
                diffusing capacity of the lung
                distolingual
                Donath-Landsteiner (test)
dl.................deciliter
DLA ....distolabial
DLAI...........distolabioincisal
DLCO ....diffusing capacity of the lung for carbon monoxide

DLE ....discoid lupus erythematosus
disseminated lupus erythematosus
DLI ....distolinguoincisal
DLO ....distolinguo-occlusal
DLP............distolinguopulpal
DM ....diabetes mellitus
diabetic mother
diastolic murmur
dopamine
DMA............dimethyladenosine
DMAB ....dimethylaminobenzaldehyde
DMBA ....dimethylbenzanthracene
DMCT..........demethylchlortetracycline
DMD............Doctor of Medical Dentistry
Duchenne's muscular dystrophy
DME............dimethyl ether (of *d*-tubocurarine)
Director of Medical Education
DMF............decayed, missing, or filled (teeth)
DMH............Department of Mental Health
DMM ....dimethylmyleran
DMN............dimethylnitrosamine
DMO............dimethyloxazolidinedione
DMPA..........depomedroxyprogesterone acetate
DMPE..........dimethoxyphenylethylamine
DMPEA ....dimethoxyphenylethylamine
DMPP..........dimethylphenylpiperazinium
DMS ....Department of Medicine and Surgery
dimethylsulfoxide
DMSO..........dimethylsulfoxide
DMT ....dimethyltryptamine
DN ....dextrose-nitrogen (ratio)
DNA ....deoxyribonucleic acid
DNase..........deoxyribonuclease
DNB ....dinitrobenzene
Diplomate of the National Board of Medical Examiners
DNC ....dinitrocarbanilide
DNCB..........dinitrochlorobenzene
DND............died a natural death
DNFB..........dinitrofluorobenzene
DNP ....deoxyribonucleoprotein
dinitrophenol

DNPH..........dinitrophenylhydrazine
DNPM.........dinitrophenylmorphine
DNT............did not test
DO...............diamine oxidase
                disto-occlusal
                Doctor of Osteopathy
DOA............dead on arrival
DOB............date of birth
DOC............deoxycholate
                deoxycorticosterone
                died of other causes
                doctor
DOCA..........deoxycorticosterone acetate
DOCS..........deoxycorticoids
DOD............date of death
                dead of disease
DOE............dyspnea on exercise
                dyspnea on exertion
DOET..........dimethoxyethyl amphetamine
DOM............deaminated-*O*-methyl metabolite
                dimethoxymethyl amphetamine
DOMA.........dihydroxymandelic acid
DON............diazo-oxonorleucine
DONEC ALV SOL FUERIT...until the bowels are open (*donec alvus soluta fuerit*)
DOPA..........dihydroxyphenylalanine
DOPAC........dihydroxyphenylacetic acid
DOS.............Division of Operational Safety
DOT.............Department of Transportation
DP...............dementia praecox
                diastolic pressure
                directional preponderance
                disability pension
                distopulpal
                Doctor of Pharmacy
                Doctor of Podiatry
                with proper direction
DPA............dipropylacetate
DPC............delayed primary closure
DPD............diffuse pulmonary disease

DPG ....diphosphoglycerate
            displacement placentogram
DPGM..........diphosphoglyceromutase
DPGP ....diphosphoglycerate phosphatase
DPH ....diphenylhydantoin
            Diploma in Public Health
DPHN..........Department of Public Health Nursing
DPI ....disposable personal income
DPL.............distopulpolingual
DPM............Diploma in Psychological Medicine
            Doctor of Podiatric Medicine
dpm ....disintegrations per minute
DPN ....diphosphopyridine nucleotide
DPNH..........diphosphopyridine nucleotide
DPO ....dimethoxyphenyl penicillin
DPS.............dimethylpolysiloxane
DPSC ....Defense Personnel Support Center
DPT.............diphtheria, pertussis, and tetanus
            dipropyltryptamine
DPTA ....diethylenetriamine pentaacetic acid
DQ ....developmental quotient
DR. ....diabetic retinopathy
            doctor
            reaction of degeneration
dr ....drachm
            dram
DRF ....Deafness Research Foundation
            dose-reduction factor
DRI ....Discharge Readiness Inventory
DS...............dead space
            dehydroepiandrosterone sulfate
            dextrose-saline
            Down's syndrome
            dry swallow
D&S ....dermatology and syphilology
DSAP ....disseminated superficial actinic porokeratosis
DSC.............disodium cromoglycate
            Doctor of Surgical Chiropody
DSCG ....disodium cromoglycate
DSM ....dextrose solution mixture
            Diagnostic and Statistical Manual

DST.............dexamethasone suppression test
DT...............delirium tremens
                distance test
                duration tetany
                dye test
DTBC..........*d*-tubocurarine
DTBN..........di-t-butyl nitroxide
DTC.............*d*-tubocurarine
DTD No vi ...let six such doses be given
DTM............dermatophyte test medium
DTMP..........deoxythymidine monophosphate
DTN ....diphtheria toxin normal
DTNB..........dithiobisnitrobenzoic acid
DTP.............diphtheria, tetanus, and pertussis
                distal tingling on percussion
DTPA..........diethylenetriaminepentacetic acid
DTR.............deep tendon reflex
DTVM..........Diploma in Tropical Veterinary Medicine
DTZ.............diatrizoate
DU ....deoxyuridine
                diagnosis undetermined
                dog unit
                duodenal ulcer
DUMP ....deoxyuridine monophosphate
DUOD..........duodenum
DUR DOLOR...while the pain lasts (*durante dolore*)
DV...............double vibration
DVA ....distance visual acuity
DVM............Doctor of Veterinary Medicine
DVMS..........Doctor of Veterinary Medicine and Surgery
DVS.............Division of Vital Statistics
                Doctor of Veterinary Science
                Doctor of Veterinary Surgery
DVSM..........Diploma in Veterinary State Medicine
DW..............distilled water
                dry weight
D/W.............dextrose in water
D-5-W..........5 per cent dextrose in water
D₅W.............5 per cent dextrose in water

DX...............dextran
                     diagnosis
DXD............discontinued
DXM............dexamethasone
DXT............deep x-ray therapy
DZ...............dizygous

E

E ....cortisone (compound E)
electric charge
electromotive force
electron
emmetropia
energy
Entamoeba
epinephrine
Escherichia
experimenter
eye
from
EA...............each
ethacrynic acid
EAC ....Ehrlich ascites carcinoma
external auditory canal
EACA..........epsilon aminocaproic acid
EAD ....the same (*eadem*)
EAE ....experimental allergic encephalomyelitis
EAHF..........eczema, asthma, hay fever
EAHLG........equine antihuman lymphoblast globulin
EAHLS ....equine antihuman lymphoblast serum
EAM............external auditory meatus
EAP.............epiallopregnanolone
EAR ....reaction of degeneration
EB...............elementary body
epidermolysis bullosa
Epstein-Barr (virus)
estradiol benzoate
EBI ....emetine bismuth iodide
EBV ....Epstein-Barr virus
EC...............electron capture
enteric-coated
entrance complaint
Escherichia coli
excitation-contraction
extracellular
eyes closed

ECA ....ethacrynic acid
ECBV ....effective circulating blood volume
ECF.............effective capillary flow
                extended care facility
                extracellular fluid
ECFMG ....Education Council for Foreign Medical Graduates
ECFV ....extracellular fluid volume
ECG ....electrocardiogram
ECHO..........Electronic Computing Hospital Oriented
                enteric cytopathogenic human orphan (virus)
                Evidence for Community Health Organization
ECI ....extracorporeal irradiation (of blood)
ECIB...........extracorporeal irradiation of blood
ECIL ....extracorporeal irradiation of lymph
ECLEC........eclectic
ECLT...........euglobulin clot lysis time
ECM ....extracellular material
ECS.............electroconvulsive shock
ECT.............electroconvulsive therapy
ECV ....extracellular volume
ECW............extracellular water
ED...............effective dose
                Ehlers-Danlos syndrome
                epileptiform discharge
                erythema dose
ED_{50} ....median effective dose
EDC ....estimated date of confinement
                expected date of confinement
EDD ....effective drug duration
                expected date of delivery
EDP ....electronic data processing
                end-diastolic pressure
EDS.............Ehlers-Danlos syndrome
EDTA ....edetic acid
                ethylenediamine tetraacetic acid
EDV ....end-diastolic volume
EE...............Eastern equine encephalitis
                end to end
                eye and ear
EEA ....electroencephalic audiometry

EEC ....enteropathogenic Escherichia coli
EEE ....Eastern equine encephalitis
EEG ....electroencephalogram
EEME..........ethinylestradiol methyl ether
EENT ....eye, ear, nose, and throat
EER ....electroencephalic response
EF ....ectopic focus
                ejection fraction
                encephalitogenic factor
EFA.............Epilepsy Foundation of America
                essential fatty acids
                extrafamily adoptees
EFC.............endogenous fecal calcium
EFE.............endocardial fibroelastosis
EFV.............extracellular fluid volume
EFVC ....expiratory flow-volume curve
EG...............esophagogastrectomy
EGG ....electrogastrogram
EGL.............eosinophilic granuloma of the lung
EGM ....electrogram
EGOT ....erythrocyte glutamic oxaloacetic transaminase
EH...............essential hypertension
EHBF..........estimated hepatic blood flow
                exercise hyperemia blood flow
EHC ....enterohepatic circulation
                essential hypercholesterolemia
EHDP..........ethane hydroxydiphosphate
EHF ....exophthalmos-hyperthyroid factor
EHL ....endogenous hyperlipidemia
EHO ....extrahepatic obstruction
EHP ....excessive heat production
EHS.............Emergency Health Services
EI................enzyme inhibitor
E/I...............expiration-inspiration ratio
EID ....egg infective dose
                electroimmunodiffusion
EIP.............extensor indicis proprius
EK...............erythrokinase
EKC ....epidemic keratoconjunctivitis
EKG ....electrocardiogram

EKY ....electrokymogram
EL................elixir
ELB ....elbow
ELIX ....elixir
ELT.............euglobulin lysis time
EM ....ejection murmur
               electron microscopy
               emmetropia
               erythrocyte mass
EMB............embryology
               eosin methylene blue
               ethambutol
               ethambutol-myambutol
EMC............electron microscopy
               encephalomyocarditis
EMF ....electromagnetic flowmeter
               electromotive force
               endomyocardial fibrosis
               erythrocyte maturation factor
EMG............electromyogram
               exophthalmos, macroglossia, gigantism
EMP ....a plaster (*emplastrum*)
               as directed
EMT ....Emergency Medical Technician
EMUL..........emulsion
EN................enema
               erythema nodosum
ENA ....extractable nuclear antigen
ENEM ....enema
ENG ....electronystagmograph
ENL ....erythema nodosum leproticum
ENT.............ear, nose, and throat
EO................eosinophils
               ethylene oxide
               eyes open
EOD ....entry on duty
               every other day
EOG ....electro-oculogram
EOM............extraocular movements
EOS.............eosinophils

EOT.............effective oxygen transport
EP...............ectopic pregnancy
              erythrocyte protoporphyrin
EPC.............epilepsia partialis continua
EPEC ....enteropathogenic Escherichia coli
EPF.............exophthalmos-producing factor
EPI.............epinephrine
EPP.............erythropoietic protoporphyria
EPR.............electron paramagnetic resonance
              electrophrenic respiration
              estradiol production rate
EPS.............exophthalmos-producing substance
EPTE..........existed prior to enlistment
EPTS..........existed prior to service
Eq ....equivalent
ER...............ejection rate
              emergency room
              endoplasmic reticulum
              external resistance
              evoked response
ERA ....evoked response audiometry
ERBF ....effective renal blood flow
ERF.............Education and Research Foundation
ERG ....electroretinogram
ERP.............effective refractory period
              equine rhinopneumonitis
ERPF ....effective renal plasma flow
ERS.............Economic Research Service
              Emergency Room Service
ERV ....expiratory reserve volume
ES ....end to side
              Expectation Score
ESB.............electrical stimulation to the brain
ESC.............electromechanical slope computer
ESCH ....Escherichia
ESD.............electronic summation device
ESE.............electrostatic unit
ESF.............erythropoietic-stimulating factor
ESL.............end-systolic length
ESM ....ejection systolic murmur

ESO..............esophagoscopy
                esophagus
ESP..............end-systolic pressure
                extrasensory perception
ESR..............erythrocyte sedimentation rate
ESS..............erythrocyte-sensitizing substance
                essential
ESS NEG.....essentially negative
EST..............electroshock therapy
                estimated
ESU..............electrostatic unit
ESV..............end-systolic volume
ET...............and
                effective temperature
                ejection time
                endotracheal
                etiology
                ethyl
                eustachian tube
ET AL..........and others (*et alii*)
ETA..............ethionamide
ETH..............elixir terpin hydrate
ETH/C.........elixir terpin hydrate with codeine
ETIOL.........etiology
ETM............erythromycin
ETOH..........ethyl alcohol
ETOX..........ethylene oxide
ETP..............entire treatment period
                eustachian tube pressure
ETT..............extrathyroidal thyroxine
ETU..............Emergency Treatment Unit
ETV..............educational television
EU...............Ehrlich units
                enzyme units
EV...............extravascular
ev...............electron volt
EVAL..........evaluation
EW...............elsewhere
                Emergency Ward

EWB............estrogen withdrawal bleeding
EWL............egg-white lysozyme
EX...............excision
               exophthalmos
               from
EXAM..........examination
EXBF..........exercise hyperemia blood flow
EXC ....excision
EXHIB ....let it be given (*exhibeatur*)
EXP.............expired
EXPIR.........expiratory
EXT............exterior
               external
               extract
               spread (*extende*)

F

F	Fahrenheit
	fat
	father
	fellow
	female
	field of vision
	Filaria
	foramen
	formula
	French (catheter size)
	Fusiformis
	gilbert (unit of magnetomotive force)
	hydrocortisone (compound F)
	make (*fiat*)
F_1	first filial generation
F_2	second filial generation
F PIL	let pills be made (*fiant pilulae*)
F VS	let the patient be bled (*fiat venaesectio*)
FA	far advanced
	fatty acid
	femoral artery
	field ambulance
	first aid
	fluorescent antibody
	forearm
	free acid
FACA	Fellow of the American College of Anesthesiologists
FACD	Fellow of the American College of Dentists
FACHA	Fellow of the American College of Hospital Administrators
FACOG	Fellow of the American College of Obstetrics and Gynecology
FACP	Fellow of the American College of Physicians
FACR	Fellow of the American College of Radiology
FACS	Fellow of the American College of Surgeons
FAD	flavin adenine dinucleotide
FADF	fluorescent antibody darkfield
FAHR	Fahrenheit

FAM DOC ...family doctor
FAMA..........Fellow of the American Medical Association
FAN ....fuchsin, amido black, and naphthol yellow
FAO.............Food and Agriculture Organization
FAPHA........Fellow of the American Public Health Association
FAR.............faradic
FASEB ....Federation of American Societies for Experimental
                 Biology
FAT.............fluorescent antibody test
FAV.............feline ataxia virus
FB...............fingerbreadth
                 foreign body
FBE ....full blood examination
FBP.............femoral blood pressure
                 fibrinogen breakdown products
FBS.............fasting blood sugar
                 fetal bovine serum
FC...............finger clubbing
                 finger counting
FCA.............ferritin-conjugated antibodies
FCC.............Federal Communications Commission
FCDA..........Federal Civil Defense Administration
FCG.............French catheter gauge
FD...............fatal dose
                 focal distance
                 foot drape
                 forceps delivery
                 freeze-dried
FD$_{50}$.............median fatal dose
FDA ....Food and Drug Administration
                 frontodextra anterior
FDE ....final drug evaluation
FDP.............fibrin degradation product
                 frontodextra posterior
                 fructose 1, 6-diphosphate
FDT.............frontodextra transversa
FEB DUR ...while the fever lasts (*febre durante*)
FEC.............free erythrocyte coproporphyrin
FECG ....fetal electrocardiogram
FECP ....free erythrocyte coproporphyria
FECVC........functional extracellular fluid volume

FEF............forced expiratory flow
FEKG..........fetal electrocardiogram
FEM...........female
FEP............Federal Employees Program
            free erythrocyte protoporphyrin
FEPP..........free erythrocyte protoporphyrin
FES............forced expiratory spirogram
FET............forced expiratory time
FETS..........forced expiratory time, in seconds
FEV............forced expiratory volume
FF..............fat free
            father factor
            fecal frequency
            filtration fraction
            finger to finger
            flat feet
            force fluids
            forearm flow
            foster father
FFA............free fatty acids
FFDW..........fat-free dry weight
FFM...........fat-free mass
FFP............fresh frozen plasma
FFT............flicker fusion threshold
FFWW.........fat-free wet weight
FG.............fibrinogen
FGD...........fatal granulomatous disease
FGF...........father's grandfather
            fresh gas flow
FGM...........father's grandmother
FH.............family history
            fetal head
            fetal heart
            let a draught be made (*fiat haustus*)
FHR...........fetal heart rate
FHT...........fetal heart
            fetal heart tones
FI..............fever caused by infection
            fibrinogen
FIB............fibrillation
            fibrinogen

FICD ....Fellow of the International College of Dentists
FICS...........Fellow of the International College of Surgeons
FID ....flame ionization detector
FIF..............forced inspiratory flow
FIG..............figure
FIGLU ....formiminoglutamic acid
FIGO ....International Federation of Gynecology and Obstetrics
FILT............filter
FIST...........fistula
FJN ....familial juvenile nephrophthisis
FL ....fluid
fl dr ....fluid dram
fl oz..............fluid ounce
FL UP ....flare-up
follow-up
FLA..............according to rule (*fiat lege artis*)
frontolaeva anterior
FLD..............fluid
FLEX ....Federal Licensing Examination
FLOR ....flowers
FLP..............frontolaeva posterior
FLSA...........follicular lymphosarcoma
FLT ....frontolaeva transversa
FM ....flowmeter
make a mixture (*fiat mistura*)
FME ....full-mouth extraction
FMF ....familial Mediterranean fever
FMG ....foreign medical graduate
FMN............flavin mononucleotide
FMS ....fat-mobilizing substance
full-mouth series
FN...............false-negative
finger to nose
FNB ....Food and Nutrition Board
FNIF ....Florence Nightingale International Foundation
FO...............foramen ovale
fronto-occipital
FOAVF........failure of all vital forces
FOD ....free of disease

FOL............leaves (*folia*)
FORE ....Foundation of Record Education
FP ....false-positive
family practice
Family Practitioner
freezing point
frontoparietal
frozen plasma
let a potion be made (*fiat potio*)
FPA............fluorophenylalanine
FPC............fish protein concentrate
FPM ....filter paper microscopic (test)
fps...............frames per second
FR...............Fisher-Race (notation)
flocculation reaction
French (catheter gauge)
FR BB ....fracture of both bones
F&R ....force and rhythm
FRACT DOS...in divided doses (*fracta dosi*)
FRAG ....fragility
FRC............frozen red cells
functional reserve capacity
functional residual capacity
FRCP ....Fellow of the Royal College of Physicians
FRCP(C)......Fellow of the Royal College of Physicians of Canada
FRCS...........Fellow of the Royal College of Surgeons
FRCS(C) ......Fellow of the Royal College of Surgeons of Canada
FRCVS ....Fellow of the Royal College of Veterinary Surgeons
FROM..........full range of motion
FRP............functional refractory period
FRS ....Fellow of the Royal Society
furosemide
FS ....full scale (IQ)
function study
FSA.............let it be made skillfully (*fiat secundum artem*)
FSD............focus to skin distance
FSF ....fibrin-stabilizing factor
FSH............follicle-stimulating hormone
FSMB ....Federation of State Medical Boards
FSP ....fibrinogen-split products
fibrinolytic split products
FS&Q ....Functions, Standards, and Qualifications

FSTPP.........Foreign Service Team Preceptorship Program
FSW ....Field Social Worker
FT ....false transmitter
              family therapy
              fibrous tissue
              free thyroxine
              full term
              make (*fiat*)
ft..................foot
FT MAS DIV IN PIL...make a mass and divide into pills (*fiat massa dividenda in pilulae*)
FT PULV .....make a powder (*fiat pulvis*)
FTA.............fluorescent treponemal antibody
FTA-AB ....fluorescent treponemal antibody absorption test
FTA-ABS .....fluorescent treponemal antibody absorption test
FTC.............Federal Trade Commission
FTI..............free thyroxine index
FTT ....failure to thrive
FU...............fecal urobilinogen
              fluorouracil
              follow-up
FUDR..........fluorodeoxyuridine
FUO ....fever of undetermined origin
              fever of unknown origin
FUR ....fluorouracil riboside
FV ....fluid volume
FVC.............forced vital capacity
FVE.............forced expiratory volume
FVL.............femoral vein ligation
FW ....Felix-Weil (reaction)
              Folin and Wu's (method)
              fragment wound
FWR...........Felix-Weil reaction
FX...............fracture
              frozen section
FY ....fiscal year
FYI..............for your information

G

G	an immunoglobulin
	force (the pull of gravity)
	gauge
	gingival
	gonidial colony
	good
	gravida
	Greek
g	gram
GA	Gamblers Anonymous
	gastric analysis
	general anesthesia
	gestational age
	gingivoaxial
	glucuronic acid
	gut-associated
GABA	gamma-aminobutyric acid
gal	gallon
GALT	gut-associated lymphoid tissue
GALV	galvanic
GAP	Group for the Advancement of Psychiatry
GAPD	glyceraldehyde phosphate dehydrogenase
GARG	gargle
GB	gallbladder
	Guillain-Barré syndrome
GBA	ganglionic-blocking agent
	gingivobuccoaxial
GBH	graphite-benzalkonium-heparin
GBM	glomerular basement membrane
GC	ganglion cells
	gas chromatography
	glucocorticoid
	gonococcus
	gonorrhea
	granular casts
	guanine cytosine
g-cal	gram-calorie
g-cm	gram-centimeter

63

GCS.............general clinical service
GDA ....germine diacetate
GDH ....glycerophosphate dehydrogenase
GDS.............Gradual Dosage Schedule
GE..............gastroemotional
　　　　　　　　gastroenterology
　　　　　　　　gastroenterostomy
G/E..............granulocyte-erythroid ratio
GEL QUAV...any kind of jelly (*gelatina quavis*)
GEMS..........good emergency mother substitute
GEN ....general
GET.............gastric emptying time
GET$^{1/2}$..........gastric emptying half-time
GF ....germ-free
　　　　　　　　gluten-free
　　　　　　　　grandfather
GFD ....gluten-free diet
GFR.............glomerular filtration rate
GG..............gamma globulin
GG or S........glands, goiter, or stiffness (the neck)
GGA ....general gonadotropic activity
GGG ....gamboge
GGTP..........gamma-glutamyl transpeptidase
GH..............growth hormone
GHD ....growth hormone deficiency
GHRF ....growth hormone-releasing factor
GI...............gastrointestinal
　　　　　　　　globin insulin
giga-...........one-billion
GIK ....glucose, insulin, and potassium
GIM ....gonadotropin-inhibitory material
GIS.............gas in stomach
　　　　　　　　gastrointestinal system
GIT.............gastrointestinal tract
GITT..........glucose-insulin tolerance test
GK..............glycerol kinase
GL..............gill
　　　　　　　　gland
　　　　　　　　greatest length
GLA.............gingivolinguoaxial
GLC.............gas-liquid chromatography

GLOB ....globulin
GLP.............group-living program
GLU ....glucose
GLUC ....glucose
GM ....gastric mucosa
                  general medical
                  geometric mean
                  grandmother
                  grand multiparity
gm ....gram
GMA ....glyceryl methacrylate
GMC ....general medical council
GMK...........green monkey kidney
gm-m ....gram-meter
GM&S.........general medical and surgical
GMT ....geometric mean titer
GMW ....gram-molecular weight
GN..............glomerulonephritis
                  glucose nitrogen (ratio)
                  gram-negative
GNC ....General Nursing Council
GNID..........gram-negative intracellular diplococci
GNP ....Gross National Product
GOE ....gas, oxygen, and ether
GOK ....God only knows
GOT............glutamic oxaloacetic transaminase
GP..............general paresis
                  general practice
                  general practitioner
                  glycoprotein
                  Graduate in Pharmacy
                  group (muscle)
                  guinea pig
                  gutta-percha
GPA............grade-point averages
GPAIS ....guinea pig anti-insulin serum
GPD ....glucose phosphate dehydrogenase
G6PD..........glucose-6-phosphate dehydrogenase
GPI..............general paralysis of the insane
                  glucose phosphate isomerase

GPIPID........guinea pig intraperitoneal infectious dose
GPK ....guinea pig kidney (antigen)
GPKA ....guinea pig kidney absorption test
GPM ....General Preventive Medicine
GPN ....Graduate Practical Nurse
GPS ....guinea pig serum
GPT ....glutamic pyruvic transaminase
GPUT ....galactose phosphate uridyl transferase
GR...............gastric resection
                   glutathione reductase
gr ....grains
GRA ....gonadotropin-releasing agent
GRAD ....gradually, by degrees
GRAS ....generally recognized as safe
GRAV i ....primigravida
GRF.............gonadotropin-releasing factor
GS ....general surgery
G/S ....glucose and saline
GSA.............Gross virus antigen
                   guanidinosuccinic acid
GSC.............gas-solid chromatography
                   gravity-settling culture
GSD.............genetically significant dose
                   glycogen storage disease
GSE.............gluten-sensitive enteropathy
GSH.............glomerular-stimulating hormone
                   reduced glutathione
GSR.............galvanic skin response
                   generalized Shwartzman reaction
GSSG...........oxidized glutathione
GSSR...........generalized Sanarelli-Shwartzman reaction
GSW ....gunshot wound
GT ....gingiva, treatment of
                   glucose tolerance
                   glutamyl transpeptidase
G&T.............gowns and towels
gt ....drop
GTH.............gonadotropic hormone
GTN.............glyceryl trinitrate
GTP ....glutamyl transpeptidase
                   guanosine triphosphate

GTT.............glucose tolerance test
gtt..............drops
GU...............gastric ulcer
                genitourinary
                gonococcal urethritis
GUS............genitourinary system
GV...............gentian violet
GVH ....graft versus host
GVHR.........graft-versus-host reaction
GW ....group work
GXT............graded exercise test
GYN ....gynecology
GZ...............Guilford-Zimmerman personality test

H

H ....Hauch (motile)
haustus (a draft)
height
Hemophilus
henry
high
Holzknecht unit
horizontal
hormone
hour
hypermetropia
hypo
H⁺ ....hydrogen ion
HA ....headache
height age
hemagglutinating antibody
hemagglutination
hemolytic anemia
high anxiety
hospital admission
hydroxyapatite
HAA ....hepatitis associated antigen
Hospital Activity Analysis
HABA..........hydroxybenzeneazobenzoic acid
HAD ....hemadsorption
HAHTG........horse antihuman thymus globulin
HAI ....hemagglutination inhibition
hemagglutinin inhibition
HAL ....halothane
HAP ....heredopathia atactica polyneuritiformis
histamine phosphate acid
HAPA ....hemagglutinating antipenicillin antibody
HAS.............Hospital Adjustment Scale
Hospital Administrative Services
HASHD........hypertensive arteriosclerotic heart disease
HAUST ....a draft (*haustus*)
HB ....heart block
hemoglobin
housebound

HBABA ....hydroxybenzeneazobenzoic acid
HBB ....hydroxybenzyl benzimidazole
HBD ....hydroxybutyrate dehydrogenase
HBDH ....hydroxybutyrate dehydrogenase
HBF ....hepatic blood flow
HBI ....high serum-bound iron
HBO ....hyperbaric oxygen
HBP ....high blood pressure
HBW ....high birth weight
HC................hair cell
              head compression
              hepatic catalase
              Hospital Corps
              house call
              Huntington's chorea
              hyaline casts
              hydroxycorticoid
HCC ....hydroxycholecalciferol
HCG ....human chorionic gonadotropin
HCH ....hexachlorocyclohexane
HCP ....hepatocatalase peroxidase
              hereditary coproporphyria
HCS.............Harvey Cushing Society
              human chorionic somatomammotropin
HCSM ....human chorionic somatomammotropin
HCT.............hematocrit
              homocytotrophic
              hydrochlorothiazide
HCU ....homocystinuria
HCVD ....hypertensive cardiovascular disease
HD ....at bedtime (*hora decubitus*)
              hearing distance
              heart disease
              high dosage
              Hodgkin's disease
              hydatid disease
HDBH ....hydroxybutyric dehydrogenase
HDC ....histidine decarboxylase
HDH ....heart disease history
HDL ....high density lipoprotein

HDLP ....high density lipoprotein
HDLW ....distance at which a watch is heard by the left ear
HDN ....hemolytic disease of the newborn
HDP ....hydroxydimethylpyrimidine
HDRW ....distance at which a watch is heard by the right ear
HDS ....herniated disk syndrome
HE...............human enteric
H&E ....hematoxylin and eosin
HEAT ....human erythrocyte agglutination test
HEBDOM ...a week (*hebdomada*)
HEC ....hydroxyergocalciferol
HED ....unit of roentgen-ray dosage
HEENT........head, eyes, ears, nose, and throat
HEK ....human embryo kidney
                      human embryonic kidney
HELP ....Higher Education Loan Program
                      Hospital Employees Labor Program
HEPA ....high-efficiency particulate air (filter)
HES.............Health Examination Survey
                      hydroxyethyl starch
HET.............helium equilibration time
HETP ....hexaethyltetraphosphate
HEW............Health, Education, and Welfare
HF...............Hageman factor
                      hay fever
                      heart failure
                      hemorrhagic fever
                      high flow
                      high frequency
HFI ....hereditary fructose intolerance
HFP.............hexafluoropropylene
HG...............hemoglobin
HGB ....hemoglobin
HGF ....hyperglycemic-glycogenolytic factor
HGG ....human gamma globulin
HGH ....human growth hormone
HGPRT ....hypoxanthine guanine phosphoribosyl transferase
HH ....hydroxyhexamide
HHA ....hereditary hemolytic anemia
HHB ....un-ionized hemoglobin

HHD ....hypertensive heart disease
H&Hm ....compound hypermetropic astigmatism
HHT ....hereditary hemorrhagic telangiectasia
HI................hemagglutination inhibition
                high impulsiveness
                hydroxyindole
HIA ....hemagglutination-inhibition antibody
HIAA ....hydroxyindoleacetic acid
HIBAC ....Health Insurance Benefits Advisory Council
HIC ....Health Insurance Council
HIHA...........high impulsiveness, high anxiety
HILA ....high impulsiveness, low anxiety
HIOMT ....hydroxyindole-*O*-methyl transferase
HIP ....Health Insurance Plan
HIS..............Health Interview Survey
HIT..............hemagglutination-inhibition test
                hypertrophic infiltrative tendinitis
HJ ....Howell-Jolly (bodies)
HK ....heat-killed
                heel to knee
                hexokinase
HKLM ....heat-killed Listeria monocytogenes
HL...............hearing level
                hearing loss
                histocompatibility locus
                hypermetropia, latent
H&L ....heart and lungs
HLH ....human luteinizing hormone
H-L-K ....heart, liver, kidney
HLR ....heart-lung resuscitator
HLT............human lymphocyte transformation
HLTH ....health
HLV ....herpes-like virus
HM ....hand movement(s)
                human milk
                hydatidiform mole
                manifest hypermetropia
HMD...........hyaline membrane disease
HME...........heat and moisture exchanger
HMF...........hydroxymethylfurfural

HMG............human menopausal gonadotropin
                  hydroxymethylglutaryl
HML............human milk lysozyme
HMM..........hexamethylolmelamine
HMP...........hexose monophosphate
                  hexose monophosphate pathway
                  hot moist packs
HMPG..........hydroxymethoxyphenylglycol
HMPS..........hexose monophosphate shunt
HMSAS........hypertrophic muscular subaortic stenosis
HMT............hematocrit
HN ....Head Nurse
                  hereditary nephritis
                  hilar node
                  tonight (*hac nocte*)
HN$_2$ ....nitrogen mustard, mechlorethamine
HNSHA........hereditary nonspherocytic hemolytic anemia
HO...............high oxygen
                  House Officer
                  hyperbaric oxygen
H/O..............history of
HOC ....hydroxycorticoid
HOCM ....hypertrophic obstructive cardiomyopathy
HOO ....House Officer Observer
HOOD..........hereditary osteo-onycho dysplasia
HOP ....high oxygen pressure
HOR DECUB...at bedtime (*hora decubitus*)
HOR INTERM...at intermediate hours (*horis intermediis*)
HOR SOM...at bedtime (*hora somni*)
HOR UN SPATIO...at the end of an hour (*horae unius spatio*)
HOSP ....hospital
HP...............high protein
                  House Physician
                  human pituitary
H&P ....history and physical
Hp ....haptoglobin
HPA ....hypothalamic-pituitary-adrenal
HPAA ....hydroxyphenylacetic acid
HPE ....history and physical examination
HPF.............heparin-precipitable fraction
                  high power field

HPFSH ....human pituitary follicle-stimulating hormone
HPG ....human pituitary gonadotropin
HPI ....history of present illness
HPL.............human placental lactogen
HPLA ....hydroxyphenyllactic acid
HPO ....high pressure oxygen
HPP.............hydroxypyrazolopyrimidine
HPPA ....hydroxyphenylpyruvic acid
HPPH ....hydroxyphenyl-phenylhydantoin
HPS.............Health Physics Society
                hematoxylin-phloxine-saffron
                hypertrophic pyloric stenosis
HPT.............hyperparathyroidism
HPV ....Hemophilus pertussis vaccine
HPVD ....hypertensive pulmonary vascular disease
HPVG ....hepatic portal venous gas
HR...............heart rate
                hospital record
                hospital report
                hour
H&R ....hysterectomy and radiation
Hr ....blood type factor
HRBC..........horse red blood cells
HRDI...........Hospital Reserve Disaster Inventory
HRET ....Hospital Research and Educational Trust
HRIG...........human rabies immune globulin
HRS.............Hamilton Rating Scale
                Health Resources Statistics
HRT.............heart rate
HS ....heat stable
                heme synthetase
                hereditary spherocytosis
                herpes simplex
                horse serum
                House Surgeon
                Hurler's syndrome
            ➥ on retiring (*hora somni*)
HSA.............human serum albumin
HSG.............hysterosalpingogram
HSMHA ....Health Services and Mental Health Administration

HSV.............herpes simplex virus
HT...............heart
                height
                hemagglutination titer
                Histologic Technician
                hydroxytryptamine
                hypermetropia, total
                hypertension
                hypodermic tablet
HTA.............hydroxytryptamine
HTHD..........hypertensive heart disease
HTOH..........hydroxytryptophol
HTP.............hydroxytryptophan
HTV.............herpes-type virus
HU ....hemagglutinating unit
                hydroxyurea
                hyperemia unit
HUD............Housing and Urban Affairs Department
HUS ....hemolytic-uremic syndrome
                hyaluronidase unit for semen
HUTHAS......human thymus antiserum
HV...............hepatic vein
                herpes virus
                hospital visit
H&V ....hemigastrectomy and vagotomy
HVA ....homovanillic acid
HVD ....hypertensive vascular disease
HVE ....high-voltage electrophoresis
HVH ....herpes virus hominis
HVL ....half-value layer
HVM...........high velocity missile
HVSD..........hydrogen-detected ventricular septal defect
HX...............history
HY...............hysteria
Hy ....hypermetropia
HYPO..........injection
                under
HYS.............hysteria
HZ...............Hertz

I

I ....intensity of magnetism
permanent incisor
¹³¹I ....radioactive iodine
i ....optically inactive
IA................impedance angle
internal auditory
intra-aortic
intra-arterial
IAA ....International Aerospace Abstracts
IABP...........intra-aortic balloon pumping
IAC ....internal auditory canal
IADH...........inappropriate antidiuretic hormone
IADHS.........inappropriate antidiuretic hormone syndrome
IAEA ....International Atomic Energy Agency
IAM.............internal auditory meatus
IARC ....International Agency for Research on Cancer
IAS..............interatrial septum
intra-amniotic saline infusion
IASD ....interatrial septal defect
IAT..............Independent Assessment Team
invasive activity test
iodine-azide test
IB................inclusion body
IBB ....intestinal brush border
IBC ....iron-binding capacity
IBR ....infectious bovine rhinotracheitis
IBU ....international benzoate unit
IC................inspiratory capactiy
intensive care
intercostal
intermediate care
intermittent claudication
International Classification
intracavitary
intracellular
intracerebral
intracranial
intracutaneous

IC *Continued*
     irritable colon
     isovolumic contraction
ICA ....intracranial aneurysm
ICC ....Indian childhood cirrhosis
     intensive coronary care
     Interstate Commerce Commission
     immunocompetent cells
ICCU...........intensive coronary care unit
ICD ....Institute for the Crippled and Disabled
     International Classification of Diseases
     isocitric dehydrogenase
ICDA...........International Classification of Diseases Adapted
ICDH...........isocitric dehydrogenase
ICF.............intensive care facility
     intracellular fluid
ICG ....indocyanine green
ICN ....International Council of Nurses
ICNS ....Interagency Conference on Nursing Statistics
ICRC ....International Committee of the Red Cross
ICRO ....International Cell Research Organization
ICRP ....International Commission on Radiological Protection
     tion
ICRU...........International Commission on Radiation Units
ICSH ....International Committee for Standardization in
     Haematology
     interstitial cell-stimulating hormone
ICT.............indirect Coombs' test
     inflammation of connective tissue
     insulin coma therapy
     isovolumic contraction time
ICT IND ......icterus index
ICU ....intensive care unit
ICW............intracellular water
ID...............identification
     infant deaths
     infective dose
     inside diameter
     internal diameter
     intradermal
     the same (*idem*)

I & D ....incision and drainage
ID$_{50}$.............median infective dose
IDA ....image display and analysis
                    iron deficiency anemia
IDI ....induction-delivery interval
IDM.............infant of diabetic mother
IDP ....initial dose period
IDR ....intradermal reaction
IDS.............immunity deficiency state
IDU ....idoxuridine
                    iododeoxyuridine
IDVC...........indwelling venous catheter
IE................immunizing unit
I/E...............inspiratory-expiratory ratio
IEMG...........integrated electromyogram
IEOP ....immunoelectro-osmophoresis
IEP..............immunoelectrophoresis
IF................immunofluorescence
                    interstitial fluid
                    intrinsic factor
IFA..............indirect fluorescent antibody
                    International Fertility Association
IFC..............intrinsic factor concentrate
IFMSA.........International Federation of Medical Student As-
                    sociations
IFR..............,inspiratory flow rate
IFRA ....indirect fluorescent rabies antibody (test)
IFT..............Institute of Food Technologists
IFV..............intracellular fluid volume
IG................immune globulin
                    intragastric
Ig ....immunoglobulin
IgA..............gamma A immunoglobulin
IgD..............gamma D immunoglobulin
IgE..............gamma E immunoglobulin
IgG..............gamma G immunoglobulin
IgM ....gamma M immunoglobulin
IGDM ....infant of gestational diabetic mother
IGV ....intrathoracic gas volume
IH................infectious hepatitis
                    inner half

IHA ....indirect hemagglutination
IHBTD........incompatible hemolytic blood transfusion disease
IHC ....idiopathic hypercalciuria
                  inner hair cell
IHD ....ischemic heart disease
IHF ....International Hospital Federation
IHO ....idiopathic hypertrophic osteoarthropathy
IHR ....intrinsic heart rate
IHS...............Indian Health Service
IHSA ....iodinated human serum albumin
IHSS...........idiopathic hypertrophic subaortic stenosis
IIF................indirect immunofluorescent
IJP ....internal jugular pressure
ILA...............insulin-like activity
ILB ....infant, low birth weight
ILBW ....infant, low birth weight
ILD ....ischemic leg disease
                  ischemic limb disease
IM ....infectious mononucleosis
                  internal medicine
                  intramedullary
                  intramuscular
im-...............(indicates presence of) NH group
IMA.............Industrial Medical Association
                  internal mammary artery
IMAA...........iodinated macroaggregated albumin
IMB.............intermenstrual bleeding
IMBC ....indirect maximum breathing capacity
IMH.............idiopathic myocardial hypertrophy
IMI..............intramuscular injection
IMP.............impression
                  improved
IMPS ....Inpatient Multidimensional Psychiatric Scale
IMR.............infant mortality rate
IMRAD ....introduction, methods, results, and discussion
IMRS ....Inpatient Multidimensional Rating Scale
IMS ....incurred in military service
                  Indian Medical Service
IN................intranasal
in.................inch

INAD...........infantile neuroaxonal dystrophy
INAH...........isonicotinic acid hydrazide
INC ....increase
                   incurred
INCR...........increase
IND ....independents
                   Investigational New Drug
IN D ....daily (*in die*)
INDM ....infant of nondiabetic mother
INE ....infantile necrotizing encephalomyelopathy
INF ....inferior
                   infusion
                   pour in (*infunde*)
INFO ....information
INH ....isonicotinic acid hydrazide
INJ..............inject
INJ ENEM...let an enema be injected (*injiciatur enema*)
INL ....inlay
INOC...........inoculate
INPV ....intermittent negative-pressure assisted ventilation
INS..............idiopathic nephrotic syndrome
INT..............intermediates
                   intermittent
                   internal
IO................internal os
                   intestinal obstruction
                   intraocular
I&O ....in and out
                   intake and output
IOFB ....intraocular foreign body
IOP..............intraocular pressure
IOS..............International Organization for Standardization
IOU ....intensive therapy observation unit
IP................incisoproximal
                   incubation period
                   instantaneous pressure
                   interphalangeal
                   intraperitoneal
                   isoelectric point
IPA..............Interaction Process Analysis

I-para ....primipara
IPC..............isopropyl chlorophenyl
IPG..............impedance plethysmography
IPH ....idiopathic pulmonary hemosiderosis
IPL..............intrapleural
IPP..............intermittent positive pressure
IPPB ....intermittent positive-pressure breathing
IPPF............International Planned Parenthood Federation
IPPI ....interruption of pregnancy for psychiatric indication
IPPO ....intermittent positive-pressure inflation with oxygen
IPPR ....intermittent positive-pressure respiration
IPPV ....intermittent positive-pressure ventilation
IPRT............interpersonal reaction test
IPS..............initial prognostic score
IPU ....inpatient unit
IPV..............inactivated poliovaccine
IQ................intelligence quotient
IR................immunoreactive
                     index of response
                     internal resistance
IRBBB ....incomplete right bundle branch block
IRDS ....idiopathic respiratory distress syndrome
IRG ....immunoreactive glucagon
IRHCS.........immunoradioassayable human chorionic
                     somatomammotropin
IRHGH ....immunoreactive human growth hormone
IRI ....immunoreactive insulin
IRO ....International Refugee Organization
IRP..............International Reference Preparation
IRR ....irradiation
IRS..............infrared spectrophotometry
                     Internal Revenue Service
IRV ....inspiratory reserve volume
IS ....in situ
                     intercostal space
                     International Standard
                     interspace
ISC..............International Staging Classification
                     International Statistical Classification
                     irreversibly sickled cells

ISD..............isosorbide dinitrate
ISDN ....isosorbide dinitrate
ISF..............interstitial fluid
ISG..............immune serum globulin
ISH..............icteric serum hepatitis
ISO..............International Standards Organization
                isoproterenol
ISP..............interspace
ISR..............Institute of Surgical Research
                International Sanitary Regulations
ISRD ....International Society for the Rehabilitation of the
                Disabled
IST..............insulin sensitivity test
                insulin shock therapy
ISW ....interstitial water
IT ....implantation test
                inhalation test
                inhalation therapy
                intradermal test
                intrathecal
                intratracheal
                intratracheal tube
                intratumoral
                isomeric transition
ITLC............instant thin-layer chromatography
ITP..............idiopathic thrombocytopenic purpura
ITPA............Illinois Test of Psycholinguistic Abilities
ITT..............insulin tolerance test
ITU..............intensive therapy unit
IU................immunizing unit
                international unit
                intrauterine
IUB ....International Union of Biochemistry
IUCD...........intrauterine contraceptive device
IUD ....intrauterine death
                intrauterine device
IUDR...........iododeoxyuridine
IUFB ....intrauterine foreign body
IUGR...........intrauterine growth rate
IUM.............intrauterine fetally malnourished

IUMP...........International Union of the Medical Press
IUPAC........International Union of Pure and Applied Chemistry
IUT..............intrauterine transfusion
IV................interventricular
                 intervertebral
                 intravascular
                 intravenous
                 intraventricular
                 in vivo
                 invasive
IVAP ....in vivo adhesive platelet
IVC ....inferior vena cava
IVCC ....intravascular consumption coagulopathy
IVCD ....intraventricular conduction defect
IVCP ....inferior vena cava pressure
IVCV ....inferior venacavography
IVD ....intervertebral disk
IVF..............intravascular fluid
IVGTT ....intravenous glucose tolerance test
IVH ....intraventricular hemorrhage
IVM ....intravascular mass
IVP..............intravenous pyelogram
IVS..............interventricular septum
IVSD ....interventricular septal defect
IVT..............intravenous transfusion
IVTTT..........intravenous tolbutamide tolerance test
IVU ....intravenous urography
IWL.............insensible water loss
IWMI...........inferior wall myocardial infarction

J

J ....Joule's equivalent
                journal
JADA...........Journal of the American Dental Association
JAMA ....Journal of the American Medical Association
JBE.............Japanese B encephalitis
JCAH...........Joint Commission on Accreditation of Hospitals
JEJ.............jejunum
JG ....juxtaglomerular
JGC.............juxtaglomerular cell
JGI ....juxtaglomerular granulation index
                juxtaglomerular index
JHDA ....Junior Hospital Doctors Association
JND.............just noticeable difference
JPS.............joint position sense
JV ....jugular vein
                jugular venous
JVP ....jugular venous pulse

K

K .... absolute zero
electrostatic capacity
kathode (cathode)
Kell blood system
Kelvin
KA .... kathode
ketoacidosis
King-Armstrong (units)
KAP .... knowledge, attitudes, and practice
KAU .... King-Armstrong units
KB .... ketone bodies
KC .... kathodal closing
kc .... kilocycle
kcal .... kilocalorie
KCC .... kathodal closing contraction
KCG .... kinetocardiogram
kcps .... kilocycles per second
KCT .... kathodal closing tetanus
KD .... kathodal duration
KDT .... kathodal duration tetanus
KE .... kinetic energy
KFAB .... kidney-fixing antibody
KFS .... Klippel-Feil syndrome
kg .... kilogram
kg-cal .... kilogram-calorie
KGS .... ketogenic steroid
KHZ .... kilohertz
KIA .... Kliger iron agar
KIU .... kallikrein-inhibiting unit
KJ .... knee jerk
KK .... knee kick
KLH .... keyhole-limpet hemocyanin
KLS .... kidney, liver, spleen
KM .... kanamycin
km .... kilometer
KMV .... killed measles-virus vaccine
KN .... knee
KOC .... kathodal opening contraction
KP .... keratitic precipitates

84

KPTT...........kaolin partial thromboplastin time
KRB ....Krebs-Ringer bicarbonate buffer
KRP ....Kolmer's test with Reiter protein
                Krebs-Ringer phosphate
KS...............ketosteroid
                Klinefelter's syndrome
                Kveim-Siltzbach (test)
KSC.............kathodal closing contraction
KST.............kathodal closing tetanus
KU ....Karmen units
KUB...........kidney, ureter, and bladder
KV................killed vaccine
kv................kilovolt
kvp ....kilovolt peak
KW ....Keith-Wagener
kw ....kilowatt
KWB ....Keith, Wagener, Barker (classification)
kw-hr...........kilowatt-hour

L

L ....coefficient of induction
Lactobacillus
Latin
left
Leishmania
length
lethal
levo
ligament
light sense
liter
low
lower
lumbar
pound (*libra*)
LA ....lactic acid
left arm
left atrial
left atrium
leucine aminopeptidase
linguoaxial
local anesthesia
low anxiety
L&A ....light and accommodation
LAA ....leukocyte ascorbic acid
LAB ....laboratory
LAD ....left anterior descending
left axis deviation
LAE ....left atrial enlargement
LAF ....laminar air flow
LAG ....labiogingival
lymphangiogram
LAH ....lactalbumin hydrolysate
left atrial hypertrophy
LAI ....labioincisal
LAIT ....latex agglutination-inhibition test
LAO ....left anterior oblique
LAP ....left atrial pressure
leucine aminopeptidase

LAP *Continued*

        leukocyte alkaline phosphatase

        lyophilized anterior pituitary

LAR.............left arm recumbent

LAS.............linear alkylate sulfonate

LASER ....light amplification by stimulated emission of radiation

LAT.............lateral

LATS...........long-acting thyroid stimulator

LB...............laboratory data

        lipid body

        live births

        loose body

lb................pound (*libra*)

LBB ....left bundle branch

LBBB..........left bundle branch block

LBF.............Lactobacillus bulgaricus factor

LBI ....low serum-bound iron

LBM............lean body mass

LBNP ....lower-body negative pressure

LBW............low birth weight

LBWI ....low birth weight infant

LBWR ....lung-body weight ratio

LC ....late clamped

        lethal concentration

        lipid cytosomes

        living children

LCA.............left coronary artery

LCD ....Liquor Carbonis Detergens

LCFA ....long-chain fatty acid

LCh ....Licentiate in Surgery

LCL.............Levinthal-Coles-Lillie (bodies)

        lymphocytic lymphosarcoma

LCM ....left costal margin

        lymphatic choriomeningitis

        lymphocytic choriomeningitis

LCT.............long-chain triglyceride

LD...............labyrinthine defect

        lactic dehydrogenase

        left deltoid

LD *Continued*

              lethal dose

              light difference

              linguodistal

              living donor

              low dosage

L-D ....Leishman-Donovan (bodies)

L/D ....light-dark ratio

LD_{50} ....median lethal dose

LDA ....left dorsoanterior

              linear displacement analysis

LDD ....light-dark discrimination

LDDS ....local dentist

LDH ....lactic dehydrogenase

LDL ....loudness discomfort level

              low density lipoprotein

LDLP ....low density lipoprotein

LDP ....left dorsoposterior

LDS ....Licentiate in Dental Surgery

LDV ....lactic dehydrogenase virus

LE ....left eye

              leukoerythrogenetic

              lower extremity

              lupus erythematosus

LED ....lupus erythematosus disseminatus

LES ....local excitatory state

LET ....linear energy transfer

LF ....laryngofissure

              limit flocculation

              low forceps

LFA ....left femoral artery

              left frontoanterior

LFD ....lactose-free diet

              least fatal dose

              low forceps delivery

LFN ....lactoferrin

LFP ....left frontoposterior

LFT ....latex flocculation test

              left frontotransverse

              liver function test

LG ....large
               laryngectomy
               left gluteal
               linguogingival
LGB ....Landry-Guillain-Barré (syndrome)
LGN ....lateral geniculate nucleus
LGV.............lymphogranuloma venereum
LH...............lower half
               luteinizing hormone
LHL.............left hepatic lobe
LHRF ....luteinizing hormone-releasing factor
LI ....linguoincisal
               low impulsiveness
LIAFI ....late infantile amaurotic familial idiocy
LIB ....pound (*libra*)
LIBC ....latent iron-binding capacity
LIC MED .....Licentiate in Medicine
LIF..............left iliac fossa
LIG..............ligament
LIHA ....low impulsiveness, high anxiety
LILA ....low impulsiveness, low anxiety
LINC ....Laboratory Instrument Computer
LIQ..............liquid
               liquor
               lower inner quadrant
LIS ....lobular in situ
LK...............left kidney
LL ....left leg
               left lower
               left lung
               lower lobe
               lysolecithin
LLC.............lymphocytic leukemia
LLF ....Laki-Lorand factor
LLL.............left lower lobe
LLLI............La Leche League International
LLM ....localized leukocyte mobilization
LLQ.............left lower quadrant
LM ....light microscopy
               linguomesial

LMA ....left mentoanterior
LMD ....local medical doctor
             low molecular weight dextran
LMDX ....low molecular weight dextran
LMP ....last menstrual period
             left mentoposterior
LMS ....Licentiate in Medicine and Surgery
LMT ....left mentotransverse
LMW ....low molecular weight
LMWD ....low molecular weight dextran
LN ....lipoid nephrosis
             lupus nephritis
             lymph node
L/N ....letter-numerical (system)
LNMP ....last normal menstrual period
LNPF ....lymph node permeability factor
LO ....linguo-occlusal
             low
LOA ....leave of absence
             left occipitoanterior
LOC DOL .....to the painful spot (*loco dolenti*)
LOD ....line of duty
LOM ....limitation of motion
             loss of motion
LOP ....left occipitoposterior
LOQ ....lower outer quadrant
LOT ....left occipitotransverse
LOWBI ....low birth weight infant
LP ....latency period
             leukocyte-poor
             light perception
             linguopulpal
             lipoprotein
             low protein
             lumbar puncture
             lymphoid plasma
L/P ....lactate-pyruvate ratio
LPA ....left pulmonary artery
LPC ....late positive component
LPE ....lipoprotein electrophoresis

LPF ....leukocytosis-promoting factor
                localized plaque formation
                low power field
LPL ....lipoprotein lipase
lpm ....liters per minute
LPN ....Licensed Practical Nurse
LPO ....light perception only
LPS ....lipopolysaccharide
LPV ....left pulmonary veins
LR ....laboratory references
                lactated Ringer's solution
L/R ....left to right ratio
L&R ....left and right
L → R ....left to right
LRF ....luteinizing hormone-releasing factor
LRH ....luteinizing hormone-releasing hormone
LRQ ....lower right quadrant
LRS ....lactated Ringer's solution
LRT ....lower respiratory tract
LS ....left side
                legally separated
                liver and spleen
                lumbosacral
                lymphosarcoma
LSA ....left sacroanterior
                lymphosarcoma
LSA/RCS .....lymphosarcoma–reticulum cell sarcoma
LSB ....left sternal border
LSCA...........left scapuloanterior
LSCP...........left scapuloposterior
LSCS ....lower segment cesarean section
LSD.............lysergic acid diethylamide
LSM ....late systolic murmur
LSP ....left sacroposterior
LST ....left sacrotransverse
LSV ....left subclavian vein
LT ....left
                left thigh
                levothyroxine
                longterm
                lymphotoxin

LTB..............laryngotracheobronchitis
LTH..............lactogenic hormone
              luteotropic hormone
LT LAT........left lateral
LTPP...........lipothiamide pyrophosphate
LU...............left upper
L&U ....lower and upper
LUL.............left upper lobe
LUQ ....left upper quadrant
LV...............left ventricle
              leukemia virus
              live vaccine
LVDP ....left ventricular diastolic pressure
LVE..............left ventricular enlargement
LVEDP........left ventricular end-diastolic pressure
LVEDV........left ventricular end-diastolic volume
LVET...........left ventricular ejection time
LVF..............left ventricular failure
              low-voltage fast
              low voltage foci
LVH ....left ventricular hypertrophy
LVN ....Licensed Vocational Nurse
LVP.............left ventricular pressure
              lysine-vasopressin
LVS..............left ventricular strain
LVSP...........left ventricular systolic pressure
LVSV...........left ventricular-stroke volume
LVSW..........left ventricular stroke work
LVW............left ventricular work
LVWI...........left ventricular work index
LW ....lacerating wound
              Lee-White (method)
L/W ....living and well
L&W............living and well
LX...............local irradiation
LYMPHS .....lymphocytes
LZM ....lysozyme

M

M ....handful (*manipulus*)
      macerate
      male
      married
      Micrococcus
      Microsporum
      minute
      mix
      molar
      month
      mother
      multipara
      murmur
      muscle
      Mycobacterium
      Mycoplasma
      myopia
      strength of pole
      thousand
m ....meter
      minim
M DICT ....as directed (*moro dicto*)
M ET SIG.....mix and label (*misce et signa*)
M FT ....make a mixture (*mistura fiat*)
MA ....mandelic acid
      mean arterial (blood pressure)
      medical audit
      mental age
      Miller-Abbott (tube)
      moderately advanced
ma ....meter-angle
      milliampere
MAA ....macroaggregated albumin
MAAC..........Medical Assistance Advisory Council
MABP..........mean arterial blood pressure
MAC ....macerate
      maximum allowable concentration
      minimum alveolar concentration

MAFH..........macroaggregated ferrous hydroxide
MAGN ....large (*magnus*)
MAM ....methylazomethanol
M+AM ....myopic astigmatism
mam ....milliampere minute
MAN...........handful (*manipulus*)
               manipulate
MAN PR ......early in the morning (*mane primo*)
MANIP........manipulation
MANOVA.....multivariate analysis of variance
MAO...........maximal acid output
               monoamine oxidase
MAOI...........monoamine oxidase inhibitor
MAP ....mean aortic pressure
               mean arterial pressure
               Medical Audit Program
               megaloblastic anemia of pregnancy
               methylacetoxyprogesterone
               methylaminopurine
               muscle-action potential
MAPF..........microatomized protein food
mas..............milliampere second
MASER........microwave amplification by stimulated emission of
               radiation
               molecular application by stimulated emission of
               radiation
MASH..........Mobile Army Surgical Hospital
MATUT........in the morning
MAX...........maximum
MB ....Bachelor of Medicine
               mesiobuccal
               methylene blue
               mix well
MBA...........methylbovine albumin
MBAS..........methylene blue active substance
MBC...........maximal breathing capacity
               minimal bactericidal concentration
MBD...........methylene blue due
               minimal brain dysfunction
               Morquio-Brailsford disease

MBF............myocardial blood flow
MBFLB ....monaural bifrequency loudness balance
MBL............minimal bactericidal level
MBO............mesiobucco-occlusal
MBP............antigen prepared from melitensis
            mean blood pressure
            mesiobuccopulpal
MBSA..........methylated bovine serum albumin
MC ....mast cell
            Master of Surgery
            maximum concentration
            Medical Corps
            Medicare
            megacurie
            megacycle
            metacarpal
            mineralocorticoid
            myocarditis
            mytomycin-C
MC P S........megacycles per second
mc ....millicurie
MCA............methylcholanthrene
MCAT..........Medical College Admission Test
            Medical College Aptitude Test
MCB............membranous cytoplasmic body
MCBR ....minimum concentration of bilirubin
MCC............mean corpuscular-hemoglobin concentration
            minimum complete-killing concentration
MCCU ....mobile coronary care unit
MCD............mean cell diameter
            mean corpuscular diameter
            medullary cystic disease
MCFA..........medium-chain fatty acid
mcg ....microgram
MCH............Maternal and Child Health
            mean corpuscular hemoglobin
mch ....millicurie hour
MCHC ....mean corpuscular-hemoglobin concentration
MCHR ....Medical Committee on Human Rights
MCI............mean cardiac index

MCL ....midclavicular line
　　　　　　　midcostal line
　　　　　　　most comfortable loudness level
MCP ....metacarpophalangeal
　　　　　　　mitotic-control protein
MCQ............multiple choice question
MCR............message competition ratio
　　　　　　　metabolic clearance rate
MCT ....mean circulation time
　　　　　　　mean corpuscular thickness
　　　　　　　medium-chain triglyceride
MCV ....mean clinical value
　　　　　　　mean corpuscular volume
MD ....Doctor of Medicine
　　　　　　　malic dehydrogenase
　　　　　　　manic depressive
　　　　　　　Mantoux diameter
　　　　　　　Marek's disease
　　　　　　　maternal deprivation
　　　　　　　medium dosage
　　　　　　　movement disorder
　　　　　　　muscular dystrophy
　　　　　　　myocardial damage
　　　　　　　myocardial disease
MDA............mentodextra anterior
　　　　　　　methylenedioxyamphetamine
　　　　　　　motor discriminative acuity
　　　　　　　Muscular Dystrophy Association
MDC............minimum detectable concentration
MDD............mean daily dose
MDF............mean dominant frequency
　　　　　　　myocardial depressant factor
MDH............malic dehydrogenase
MDHV ....Marek's disease herpesvirus
MDL............Master Drug List
MDM ....minor determinant mixture
MDP............mentodextra posterior
MDS ....Master of Dental Surgery
MDT............median detection threshold
　　　　　　　mentodextra transversa

MDTR	mean diameter-thickness ratio
MDUO	myocardial disease of unknown origin
MDY	month, date, year
ME	medical education
	Medical Examiner
	mercaptoethanol
	middle ear
M/E	myeloid-erythroid ratio
Me	methyl
MEA	Medical Exhibitors Association
	mercaptoethylamine
	multiple endocrine adenomatosis
MED	median
	medical
	medicine
	minimal effective dose
	minimal erythema dose
MEDLARS	Medical Literature Analysis and Retrieval System
MEDS	medications
	medicines
MEF	maximal expiratory flow
MEFR	maximum expiratory flow rate
MEG	mercaptoethylguanidine
mega-	one-million
megalo-	great size
MEM	minimum essential medium
MEP	meperidine
MEPP	miniature end-plate potential
mEq	milliequivalent
MER	mean ejection rate
	methanol-extruded residue
MESH	Medical Subject Headings
mev	million electron volts
MF	medium frequency
	mycosis fungoides
	myelin figures
M/F	male-female ratio
M&F	mother and father
Mf	microfilaria
MFB	metallic foreign body

MFC ....Master Facility Census
MFD ....midforceps delivery
                minimal fatal dose
mfd ....microfarad
MFI ....Master Facility Inventory
MFL ....Master Facility List
MFP ....monofluorophosphate
MFR ....mucus flow rate
MFW ....multiple fragment wounds
MG ....mesiogingival
                methyl glucoside
                muscle group
mg ....milligram
MGF ....mother's grandfather
MGGH ....methylglyoxal guanylhydrazone
MGH ....monoglyceride hydrolase
MGM ....mother's grandmother
mgm ....milligram
MGN ....membranous glomerulonephritis
MGP ....marginal granulocyte pool
MGR ....modified gain ratio
MGTIS ....meningitis
MH ....mammotropic hormone
                marital history
                medical history
                mental health
MHA............methemalbumin
                microangiopathic hemolytic anemia
                mixed hemadsorption
MHB............maximum hospital benefit
MHb ....methemoglobin
MHD............mean hemolytic dose
                minimum hemolytic dose
mHg ....millimeters of mercury
MHN............massive hepatic necrosis
MHP............mercurihydroxypropane
MHPG..........methoxyhydroxyphenylglycol
MHR............maximal heart rate
MI ....mercaptoimidazole
                mitral incompetence

MI *Continued*
     mitral insufficiency
     myocardial infarction
MIC..............Maternity and Infant Care
     minimum inhibitory concentration
MIC PAN.....bread crumb (*mica panis*)
micro-..........one-millionth
MICU..........mobile intensive care unit
MID..............maximum inhibiting dilution
     mesioincisodistal
     minimum infective dose
MIDNOC......midnight
MIF..............macrophage-inhibiting factor
     migration-inhibition factor
     mixed immunofluorescene
MIFR...........maximal inspiratory flow rate
milli-............one-thousandth
MIN.............minim
     minimal
     minute
min..............minim
     minute
MIO.............minimum identifiable odor
MIP.............maximum inspiratory pressure
MIRD.........medical internal radiation dose
MIRU.........myocardial infarction research unit
MIST..........mixture (*mistura*)
MIT.............monoiodotyrosine
     send (*mitte*)
MIXT..........mixture
MK..............monkey kidney
MKS...........meter-kilogram-second
MKV...........killed measles vaccine
ML..............Licentiate in Medicine
     mesiolingual
     middle lobe
     midline
M:L.............monocyte-lymphocyte ratio
ml................milliliter

MLA ....Medical Library Association
              mentolaeva anterior
              monocytic leukemia, acute
MLa.............mesiolabial
MLaI ....mesiolabioincisal
MLAP.........mean left atrial pressure
MLC ....mixed leukocyte culture
              mixed lymphocyte culture
              multilamellar cytosome
              myelomonocytic leukemia, chronic
MLD ....metachromatic leukodystrophy
              minimum lethal dose
MLI ....mesiolinguoincisal
MLO ....mesiolinguo-occlusal
MLP ....mentolaeva posterior
              mesiolinguopulpal
MLS ....mean lifespan
              myelomonocytic leukemia, subacute
MLT ....mentolaeva transversa
MLV ....Moloney's leukemogenic virus
              mouse leukemia virus
MM..............malignant melanoma
              Marshall-Marchetti
              medial malleolus
              mucous membrane
              multiple myeloma
              muscles
              muscularis mucosa
              myeloid metaplasia
M&M ....milk and molasses
mm ....millimeter
mM ....millimol
              millimolar
MMA...........methylmalonic acid
MMC ....minimal medullary concentration
MMD ....minimum morbidistatic dose
MMEF ....maximal midexpiratory flow rate
MMEFR.......maximal midexpiratory flow rate
MMF............maximal midexpiratory flow

MMFR ....maximal midexpiratory flow rate
            maximal midflow rate
mM/L...........millimols per liter
MMM...........myeloid metaplasia with myelofibrosis
            myelosclerosis with myeloid metaplasia
mmm ....micromillimeter
            millimicron
MMPI ....Minnesota Multiphasic Personality Inventory
mmpp ....millimeters partial pressure
MMPR ....methylmercaptopurine riboside
MMR ....mass miniature radiography
            mobile mass x-ray
            myocardial metabolic rate
MN..............midnight
            multinodular
            myoneural
M/N..............midnight
M&N...........morning and night
mN ....millinormal
MNA............maximum noise area
MNCV ....motor nerve conduction velocity
MNU............methylnitrosourea
MO ....Medical Officer
            mesio-occlusal
            mineral oil
            month
MOD............mesio-occlusodistal
            moderate
MOD PRAESC ...in the way directed (*modo praescripto*)
MOH............Medical Officer of Health
MOL WT ......molecular weight
MOLL..........soft (*mollis*)
MOM ....milk of magnesia
MOMA ....methoxyhydroxymandelic acid
MOPV..........monovalent oral poliovirus vaccine
MOR DICT...in the manner directed (*more dicto*)
MOR SOL.....in the usual way (*more solito*)
MORC..........Medical Officers Reserve Corps
mOs ....milliosmolal
mOsm ....milliosmol

MP ....as directed (*modo prescripto*)
               mean pressure
               melting point
               menstrual period
               mercaptopurine
               mesiopulpal
               metacarpophalangeal
               monophosphate
               mucopolysaccharide
               multiparous
MPA ....main pulmonary artery
               medroxyprogesterone acetate
               methylprednisolone acetate
MPAP ....mean pulmonary arterial pressure
MPC ....marine protein concentrate
               maximum permissible concentration
               meperidine, promethazine, chlorpromazine
               minimum mycoplasmacidal concentration
MPD ....maximum permissible dose
MPEH ....methylphenylethylhydantoin
MPH ....Master of Public Health
MPJ ....metacarpophalangeal joint
MPL ....mesiopulpolingual
MPLa ....mesiopulpolabial
MPN ....most probable number
MPO ....myeloperoxidase
MPP ....mercaptopyrazidopyrimidine
MPS ....mucopolysaccharide
MR ....mental retardation
               metabolic rate
               methyl red
               mitral reflux
               mitral regurgitation
               mortality rate
               mortality ratio
               muscle relaxant
mr ....milliroentgen
MRAP ....mean right atrial pressure
MRC ....Medical Research Council (units)
               Medical Reserve Corps

MRD............minimum reacting dose
MRF............mesencephalic reticular formation
 mitral regurgitant flow
MRT............median recognition threshold
 milk-ring test
MRVP..........mean right ventricular pressure
MS...............manuscript
 Master of Science
 Master of Surgery   *Miss (ms - mrs) ?;*
 mental status
 mitral stenosis
 morphine sulfate
 mucosubstance
 multiple sclerosis
 musculoskeletal
MSA............Medical Services Administration
msec............millisecond
MSER..........mean systolic ejection rate
MSG............monosodium glutamate
MSH............medical self-help
 melanocyte-stimulating hormone
 melanophore-stimulating hormone
MSHFA........Multiservice Health Facility Association
MSK............medullary sponge kidney
MSL............midsternal line
MSLA..........mouse-specific lymphocyte antigen
MSN............mildly subnormal
MSRPP........multidimensional scale for rating psychiatric pa-
 tients
MSS.............mental status schedule
MSU............monosodium urate
MSUD..........maple syrup urine disease
MSV............Moloney sarcoma virus
 murine sarcoma virus
MSW............Master of Social Work
MT...............empty
 malignant teratoma
 maximal therapy
 medical technologist
 membrana tympani

MT *Continued*
    metatarsal
    methyltyrosine
    more than
    music therapy
MTD ....maximum tolerated dose
MTDT ....modified tone decay test
MTF ....maximum terminal flow
    modulation transfer function
MTHF ....methyltetrahydrofolic acid
MTI ....malignant teratoma intermediate
    minimum time interval
MTN ....Medical Television Network
MTP ....metatarsophalangeal
MTR ....Meinicke turbidity reaction
MTT............malignant teratoma trophoblastic
    monotetrazolium
MTU ....methylthiouracil
MTV ....mammary tumor virus
MTX ....methotrexate
MU ....Mache unit
    Montevideo unit
    mouse unit
mU ....milliunit
mu ....micron
MUC............mucilage
MULTIP ......pregnant woman who has borne children
MUST ....medical unit, self-contained, transportable
MUU............mouse uterine units
MV ....Medicus Veterinarius (veterinary physician)
    minute volume
    mitral valve
    mixed venous
mv ....millivolt
MVM............microvillose membrane
MVR............massive vitreous retraction
MVV............maximum voluntary ventilation
MW..............molecular weight
mw ....microwave

My...............myopia
my...............mayer (unit of heat capacity)
MyG.............myasthenia gravis
MZ...............monozygotic

N

N ....nasal
                Neisseria
                nerve
                neurology
                Nocardia
                normal
                unit for fast neutrons
n ....index of refraction
                size of sample
n_D ....refractive index
NA ....neutralizing antibody
                Nomina Anatomica
                noradrenaline
                not admitted
                not applicable
                not available
                numeric aperture
                Nurse Anesthetist
                Nursing Assistant
NAA ....no apparent abnormalities
NABSP ....National Association of Blue Shield Plans
NACOR ....National Advisory Committee on Radiation
NAD ....nicotinamide adenine dinucleotide
                no appreciable disease
                normal axis deviation
NADH ....nicotinamide adenine dinucleotide (reduced form)
NADP ....nicotinamide adenine dinucleotide phosphate
NADPH ....nicotinamide adenine dinucleotide phosphate
                (reduced form)
NAME ....National Association of Medical Examiners
NAMH ....National Association of Mental Health
NANA ....*N*-acetylneuraminic acid
nano- ....one-billionth
NAPA ....*N*-acetyl-*p*-aminophenol
NAPCA ....National Air Pollution Control Administration
NAPNE ....National Association for Practical Nurse Education
NAPPH ....National Association of Private Psychiatric Hospitals
NARC ....National Association for Retarded Children
NARD ....National Association of Retail Druggists

NAS..............National Association of Sanitarians
NASA ....National Aeronautics and Space Administration
NAS-NRC.....National Academy of Sciences-National Research
                    Council
NB ....newborn
                    nitrous oxide-barbiturate
                    note well (*nota bene*)
NBM............nothing by mouth
NBME ....National Board of Medical Examiners
NBO ....nonbed occupancy
NBS ....National Bureau of Standards
                    normal burro serum
NBT ....nitroblue tetrazolium
NBTE ....nonbacterial thrombotic endocarditis
NBW ....normal birth weight
NC...............no casualty
                    no change
                    noise criterion
                    noncontributory
                    not cultured
N/C..............no complaints
nc ....nanocurie
NCA ....National Council on Alcoholism
                    neurocirculatory asthenia
NCD ....not considered disabling
NCDC..........National Communicable Disease Center
NCES ....National Center for Educational Statistics
NCHS ....National Center for Health Statistics
NCI ....National Cancer Institute
NCME ....Network for Continuing Medical Education
NCRP ....National Council on Radiation Protection
NCSH ....National Clearinghouse for Smoking and Health
ND ....neonatal death
                    neurotic depression
                    Newcastle disease
                    New Drugs
                    no data
                    no disease
                    nondisabling
                    normal delivery

ND *Continued*

        not detectable
        not detected
        not determined
        not done
NDA............National Dental Association
        New Drug Applications
        no data available
        no demonstrable antibodies
NDC............National Dairy Council
NDF............new dosage form
NDGA..........nordihydroguaiaretic acid
NDH............Natural Disaster Hospital
NDI............nephrogenic diabetes insipidus
NDMA.........nitrosodimethylaniline
NDP............net dietary protein
NDTI..........National Disease and Therapeutic Index
NDV............Newcastle disease virus
NE...............nerve ending
        neurologic examination
        no effect
        nonelastic
        norepinephrine
        not evaluated
        not examined
NEA............National Education Association
NEC............not elsewhere classifiable
        not elsewhere classified
NED............no evidence of disease
NEFA..........nonesterified fatty acid
NEG............negative
NEM............*N*-ethylmaleimide
NEMA.........National Eclectic Medical Association
NE TR S NUM...do not deliver unless paid (*ne tradas sine nummo*)
NEURO.......neurologic
NEUROL.....neurologic
NF...............National Formulary
        none found
        normal flow
        not found

NFLPN........National Federation of Licensed Practical Nurses
NFPA..........National Fire Protection Association
NFTD..........normal full-term delivery
NG...............nasogastric
ng................nanogram
NGF.............nerve growth factor
NGO............Nongovernmental Observer
NGU............nongonococcal urethritis
NH..............nonhuman
               nursing home
NHA............nonspecific hepatocellular abnormality
NHC............National Health Council
NHI.............National Health Insurance
               National Heart Institute
NHLI...........National Heart and Lung Institute
NHMRC.......National Health and Medical Research Council
NHS............National Health Service
               normal horse serum
               normal human serum
NI................no information
               not identified
               not isolated
NIA.............no information available
NIAID.........National Institute of Allergy and Infectious Diseases
NIAMD........National Institute of Arthritis and Metabolic Diseases
NICHHD......National Institute of Child Health and Human Development
NIDR...........National Institute of Dental Research
NIEHS.........National Institute of Environmental Health Sciences
NIGMS........National Institute of General Medical Sciences
NIH.............National Institutes of Health
NIL.............none
NIMH..........National Institute of Mental Health
NIMP...........National Intern Matching Program
NINDB........National Institute of Neurological Diseases and Blindness
NINDS.........National Institute of Neurological Diseases and Stroke
NIRMP........National Intern and Resident Matching Program

NK ....not known
NKH ....nonketotic hyperosmotic
Nl ....normal
NLA ....neuroleptanalgesia
NLM ....National Library of Medicine
NLN ....National League for Nursing
NLNE ....National League of Nursing Education
NLT ....normal lymphocyte transfer test
NM ....neuromuscular
                not measurable
                not measured
                not mentioned
                nuclear medicine
Nm ....nutmeg
nm ....nanometer
NMA ....National Medical Association
                neurogenic muscular atrophy
NMAC ....National Medical Audiovisual Center
NMP ....normal menstrual period
NMRI ....Naval Medical Research Institute
N:N ....(indicates presence of) the azo group
nn ....nerves
NND ....neonatal death
                New and Nonofficial Drugs
NNI ....noise and number index
NNN ....Nicolle-Novy-MacNeal (medium)
NNR ....New and Nonofficial Remedies
NO ....none obtained
No ....number
NOA ....Nurse Obstetric Assistant
NOC ....night
NOCT ....at night (*nocte*)
NOCT MANEQ...at night and in the morning (*nocte maneque*)
NON-REM ...nonrapid eye movement
NON REP.....do not repeat (*non repetatur*)
NON REPETAT...do not repeat (*non repetatur*)
NOPHN........National Organization for Public Health Nursing
NOS.............not otherwise specified
NOSIE.........Nurses Observation Scale for Inpatient Evaluation
NOTB ....National Ophthalmic Treatment Board (British)

NP...............nasopharyngeal
nasopharynx
neuropathology
neuropsychiatric
normal plasma
not performed
nucleoplasmic index
nucleoprotein
nursing procedure
NPA ....National Pituitary Agency
NPB ....nodal premature beat
NPC ....near point of convergence
NPD ....Niemann-Pick disease
NPH ....neutral protamine Hagedorn (insulin)
NPN ....nonprotein nitrogen
NPO ....nothing by mouth (*nulla per os*)
NPO/HS ....nothing by mouth at bedtime (*nulla per os hora somni*)
NPT.............neoprecipitin test
NPU ....net protein utilization
NR...............do not repeat (*non repetatur*)
no radiation
no response
nonreactive
normal
not readable
not recorded
not resolved
NRBC..........nucleated red blood cell
NRC ....National Research Council
normal retinal correspondence
NRD ....nonrenal death
NRDC..........National Respiratory Disease Conference
NREM ....nonrapid eye movement
NRS.............normal rabbit serum
normal reference serum
NS ....nephrotic syndrome
nervous system
neurologic survey
no sample

NS *Continued*
               no specimen
               nonspecific
               nonsymptomatic
               normal saline
               not significant
               not sufficient
N/S .... normal saline
NSA .... no serious abnormality
               no significant abnormality
NSC .... no significant change
               not service-connected
NSCD .... nonservice-connected disability
NSD .... no significant defect
               no significant deviation
               no significant difference
               no significant disease
               normal spontaneous delivery
NSDP .... National Society of Denture Prosthetists
NSF .... National Science Foundation
NSG .... nursing
NSM .... neurosecretory material
NSMR .... National Society for Medical Research
NSND .... nonsymptomatic, nondisabling
NSPB .... National Society for the Prevention of Blindness
NSQ .... not sufficient quantity
NSR .... normal sinus rhythm
NSS .... normal saline solution
               not statistically significant
NSU .... nonspecific urethritis
NT .... nasotracheal
               neutralization test
               neutralizing
               nontypable
               not tested
NTA .... National Tuberculosis Association
NTAB .... nephrotoxic antibody
NTG .... nontoxic goiter
NTN .... nephrotoxic nephritis
NTP .... normal temperature and pressure

NTRDA........National Tuberculosis and Respiratory Disease Association
NTRS...........National Therapeutic Recreation Society
NV...............negative variation
N&V............nausea and vomiting
Nv...............naked vision
NVA............near visual acuity
NWB...........no weight bearing
NYD............not yet diagnosed
NYHA..........New York Heart Association (classification)

O

O .... eye (*oculus*)
                none
                nonmotile
                obstetrics
                opening
                oral
                orderly
                pint (*octarius*)
                respirations (anesthesia chart)
                suture size
O_2 .... both eyes
                oxygen
O_2 CAP .... oxygen capacity
O M .... every morning (*omni mane*)
O N .... every night (*omni nocte*)
O- .... ortho
OA .... osteoarthritis
                oxalic acid
OAA .... Old Age Assistance
OAAD .... ovarian ascorbic acid depletion
OAD .... obstructive airway disease
OAP .... osteoarthropathy
OAR .... other administrative reasons
OASI .... Old Age and Survivors Insurance
OB .... objective benefit
                obstetrics
O&B .... opium and belladonna
OBG .... obstetrics and gynecology
OBL .... oblique
OBS .... obstetrical service
                obstetrics
                organic brain syndrome
OBST .... obstetrics
OC .... occlusocervical
                office call
                on call
                oral contraceptive
                original claim
OCC .... occasional

OCHAMPUS...Office for the Civilian Health and Medical Program
for the Uniformed Services
OCR ....optical character recognition
OCT............ornithine carbamyl transferase
OCV ....ordinary conversational voice
OD...............Doctor of Optometry
Officer of the Day
once a day
optical density
outside diameter
overdose
od ....right eye (*oculus dexter*)
ODA ....occipitodextra anterior
ODM............ophthalmodynamometry
ODMC ....Office for Dependents Medical Care
ODP ....occipitodextra posterior
ODT............occipitodextra transversa
O&E ....observation and examination
OEF............oil emersion field
OEO ....Office of Economic Opportunity
OER ....oxygen enhancement ratio
OF...............Ovenstone factor
Of................official
OFC............occipitofrontal circumference
OFD ....oral-facial-digital
OG...............obstetrics and gynecology
O&G ....obstetrics and gynecology
OGS............oxogenic steroid
OGTT...........oral glucose tolerance test
OH...............occupational history
OHC ....outer hair cell
OHCS ....hydroxycorticosteroid
OHP ....oxygen under high pressure
OIH ....orthoiodohippurate
OJ................orange juice
OKN ....optokinetic nystagmus
OL ....left eye
Ol................oil
Ol res ....oleoresin
OLA............occipitolaeva anterior

OLH ....ovine lactogenic hormone
OLP............occipitolaeva posterior
OL&T ....owners, landlords, and tenants
OM ....Occupational Medicine
               otitis media
OMD............ocular muscle dystrophy
OMI............old myocardial infarction
OMN BIH.....every two hours (*omni bihora*)
OMN HOR ...every hour (*omni hora*)
OMN NOCT..every night (*omni nocte*)
OMPA..........octamethylpyrophosphoramide
OM QUAR HOR...every quarter of an hour (*omni quarta hora*)
OOB ....out of bed
OP...............opening pressure
               operation
               osmotic pressure
               outpatient
O&P ....ova and parasites
OPC............Outpatient Clinic
OPD ....Outpatient Department
OPG............oxypolygelatin
OPH ....ophthalmology
OPHTH........ophthalmology
OPK ....optokinetic
OPS............Outpatient Service
OPT............outpatient
               outpatient treatment
OPV............oral poliovaccine
               oral poliovirus vaccine
OR...............operating room
ORS............orthopedic surgery
ORT............Operating Room Technician
ORTH ....orthopedics
ORTHO........orthopedics
OS ....mouth
               opening snap
               oral surgery
os ....left eye (*oculus sinister*)
OSM ....oxygen saturation meter
OST............object sorting test
               Office of Science and Technology

OT	occlusion time
	Occupational Therapist
	occupational therapy
	old term
	old terminology
	old tuberculin
	orotracheal
	otolaryngology
OTC	ornithine transcarbamylase
	over the counter
	oxytetracycline
OTD	organ tolerance dose
OTO	otolaryngology
	otology
OTOL	otology
OTR	Ovarian Tumor Registry
OU	both eyes (*oculi unitas*)
	Observation Unit
OURQ	outer upper right quadrant
OV	office visit
Ov	egg (*ovum*)
OW	out of wedlock
O/W	oil in water
	oil-water ratio
OX	oxymel
oz	ounce

P

P ....after (*post*)
              handful (*pugillus*)
              near point
              Para
              partial pressure
              Pasteurella
              pharmacopeia
              Plasmodium
              position
              postpartum
              premolar
              presbyopia
              pressure
              primipara
              protein
              Proteus
              psychiatry
              pulse
              pupil
              weight (*pondus*)
P_{NA} ....plasma sodium
P_1 ....parental generation
P_2 ....pulmonic second sound
^{32}P ....radioactive phosphorus
P AE............in equal parts (*partes aequales*)
P RAT AETAT...in proportion to age (*pro ratione aetatis*)
p................probability
p-................para
p_{CO_2} ....carbon dioxide pressure
PA...............paralysis agitans
              pathology
              per annum
              pernicious anemia
              phakic-aphakic
              Physician's Assistant
              posteroanterior
              primary amenorrhea
              primary anemia

PA *Continued*

           pulmonary artery

           pulpoaxial

P&A ....percussion and auscultation

PAB ....para-aminobenzoic acid

PABA ....para-aminobenzoic acid

PAC.............Political Action Committee

           premature auricular contraction

PAF.............pulmonary arteriovenous fistula

PAFIB ....paroxysmal atrial fibrillation

PAGMK ....primary African green monkey kidney

PAH ....para-aminohippurate

           polycyclic aromatic hydrocarbon

           pulmonary artery hypertension

PAHA ....para-aminohippuric acid

PAHO ....Pan American Health Organization

PAM............crystalline penicillin G in 2 per cent aluminum monostearate

           phenylalanine mustard

           pralidoxime chloride

           pulmonary alveolar microlithiasis

           pyridine aldoxime methiodide

PAN ....periodic alternating nystagmus

           peroxyacetyl nitrate

PANS ....puromycin aminonucleoside

PAOD ....peripheral arterial occlusive disease

           peripheral arteriosclerotic occlusive disease

PAP.............Papanicolaou (stain, smear, test)

           primary atypical pneumonia

           prostatic acid phosphatase

           pulmonary alveolar proteinosis

           pulmonary artery pressure

PAPP...........para-aminopropiophenone

PAPS...........phosphoadenosyl-phosphosulfate

PAPVC........partial anomalous pulmonary venous connection

PAR.............postanesthesia room

           pulmonary arteriolar resistance

PAR AFF.....the part affected (*pars affecta*)

PARA ....number of pregnancies

PART AEQ...equal parts (*partes aequales*)

PART VIC ...in divided doses (*partibus vicibus*)
PAS.............para-aminosalicylic acid
　　　　　periodic acid-Schiff (method, stain, technique, test)
　　　　　Professional Activity Study
　　　　　pulmonary artery stenosis
PASA...........para-aminosalicylic acid
PAS-C..........para-aminosalicylic acid crystallized with ascorbic
　　　　　acid
PASD ....after diastase digestion
　　　　　periodic acid-Schiff technique
PASM ....periodic acid-silver methenamine
Past.............Pasteurella
PAT.............paroxysmal atrial tachycardia
PATH ....pathology
PB...............Pharmacopoeia Britannica
　　　　　phenobarbital
　　　　　phonetically balanced
PBA ....pulpobuccoaxial
PBC ....prebed care
　　　　　primary biliary cirrhosis
PBF.............pulmonary blood flow
PBG ....porphobilinogen
PBI ....protein-bound iodine
PBN ....paralytic brachial neuritis
PBO............penicillin in beeswax
　　　　　placebo
PBS.............phosphate-buffered saline
PBSP...........prognostically bad signs during pregnancy
PBT$_4$............protein-bound thyroxine
PBV.............predicted blood volume
　　　　　pulmonary blood volume
PBZ.............pyribenzamine
PC.).........after meals (*post cibum*)
　　　　　per cent
　　　　　phosphate cycle
　　　　　phosphocreatine
　　　　　platelet count
　　　　　platelet concentrate
　　　　　portacaval
　　　　　pubococcygeus

PC *Continued*

               pulmonic closure

               weight (*pondus civile*)

pc ....picocurie

PCA............passive cutaneous anaphylaxis

PCB............paracervical block

PcB ....near point of convergence

PCc.............periscopic concave

PCD............phosphate-citrate-dextrose

               polycystic disease

               posterior corneal deposits

PCF............posterior cranial fossa

PCG............phonocardiogram

PCH ....paroxysmal cold hemoglobinuria

PCM ....protein-calorie malnutrition

PCMO.........Principal Colonial Medical Officer

PCN ....penicillin

pCO₂............carbon dioxide pressure

PCP............parachlorophenate

PCPA ....parachlorophenylalanine

PCPT...........perception

PCS............portacaval shunt

Pcs ....preconscious

PCT............plasmacrit

               porphyria cutanea tarda

               portacaval transposition

PCV............packed cell volume

               polycythemia vera

PCV-M.........myeloid metaplasia with polycythemia vera

PCx ....periscopic convex

PD...............Doctor of Pharmacy

               papilla diameter

               Parkinson's disease

               pediatrics

               phosphate dehydrogenase

               plasma defect

               poorly differentiated

               potential difference

               pressor dose

               prism diopter

PD *Continued*

                    progression of disease
                    psychotic depression
                    pulmonary disease
                    pulpodistal
                    pupillary distance
PDA ....patent ductus arteriosus
                    pediatric allergy
PDAB ....para-dimethylaminobenzaldehyde
PDC ....pediatric cardiology
PDD ....pyridoxine-deficient diet
PDDS ....Parasitic Disease Drug Service
PDH ....packaged disaster hospital
                    phosphate dehydrogenase
PDL..............pudendal
PDP..............piperidino-pyrimidine
PE ....pharyngoesophageal
                    phenylephrine
                    physical evaluation
                    physical examination
                    pleural effusion
                    polyethylene
                    probable error
                    pulmonary edema
                    pulmonary embolism
PEB ....Physical Evaluation Board
PEBG ....phenethylbiguanide
PED ....pediatrics
PEDS ....pediatrics
PEF..............peak expiratory flow
PEFR ....peck expiratory flow rate
PEG..............pneumoencephalography
                    polyethylene glycol
PEI..............phosphate excretion index
                    physical efficiency index
PEN ....penicillin
PENT ....pentothal
PEO..............progressive external ophthalmoplegia
PEP..............pre-ejection period
                    Psychiatric Evaluation Profile
PEPP...........positive expiratory pressure plateau

PER..............by
                    for each
                    protein efficiency ratio
                    through
PER OS ....by mouth
PERCUSS ...percussion
PERLA........pupils equal, react to light and accommodation
PERPAD......perineal pad
PERRLA......pupils equal, round, regular, react to light and
                    accommodation
PET.............pre-eclamptic toxemia
PETN ....pentaerythritol tetranitrate
PF ....personality factor
                    picture-frustration (study)
                    platelet factor
P/F ....pass-fail system
PFC.............plaque-forming cell
PFIB ....perfluoroisobutylene
PFK.............phosphofructokinase
PFO.............patent foramen ovale
PFQ.............personality factor questionnaire
PFR.............peak flow rate
PFT ....posterior fossa tumor
                    pulmonary function test
PFU.............plaque-forming units
PG...............Pharmacopoeia Germanica
                    plasma triglyceride
                    postgraduate
                    pregnant
                    prostaglandin
                    pyoderma gangrenosum
pg................picogram
PGA.............pteroylglutamic acid
PGD ....phosphogluconate dehydrogenase
                    phosphoglyceraldehyde dehydrogenase
PGDH..........phosphogluconate dehydrogenase
PGDR..........plasma-glucose disappearance rate
PGH ....pituitary growth hormone
PGI..............phosphoglucoisomerase
                    potassium, glucose, and insulin
PGK ....phosphoglycerate kinase

PGM ....phosphoglucomutase
PGP.............postgamma proteinuria
PGTR..........plasma glucose tolerance rate
PH...............past history
                personal history
                pharmacopeia
                phenyl
                prostatic hypertrophy
                public health
                pulmonary hypertension
pH ....hydrogen ion concentration
PHA ....phytohemagglutinin
PHAR..........pharmacy
PharB..........Bachleor of Pharmacy
PharC..........Pharmaceutical Chemist
PharD..........Doctor of Pharmacy
PharG..........Graduate in Pharmacy
PHARM ....pharmacy
PharM ....Master of Pharmacy
PhB.............British Pharmacopoeia
PHBB..........propylhydroxybenzyl benzimidazole
PHC ....posthospital care
PhG ....German Pharmacopeia
                Graduate in Pharmacy
PHI ....phosphohexoisomerase
                Public Health Inspector
PHK ....platelet phosphohexokinase
PHLA ....postheparin lipolytic activity
PHP.............primary hyperparathyroidism
                pseudohypoparathyroidism
PHS.............Public Health Service
PHYS ....physiology
PI................pacing impulse
                performance intensity
                pre-induction (examination)
                present illness
                protamine insulin
                Protocol Internationale
                pulmonary incompetence
                pulmonary infarction
PIA..............plasma insulin activity

pico- ....one-trillionth
PICU ....pulmonary intensive care unit
PID ....pelvic inflammatory disease
  plasma-iron disappearance
PIDT ....plasma-iron disappearance time
PIE..............pulmonary infiltration and eosinophilia
  pulmonary interstitial emphysema
PIF..............peak inspiratory flow
  prolactin-inhibiting factor
PIFR ....peak inspiratory flow rate
PII...............plasma inorganic iodine
PIL..............pill
PIP..............proximal interphalangeal
  Psychotic Inpatient Profile
PIPJ ....proximal interphalangeal joint
PIT..............plasma iron turnover
PITR...........plasma iron turnover rate
PK...............Prausnitz-Küstner (reaction)
  psychokinesis
  pyruvate kinase
PKU ....phenylketonuria
PKV ....killed poliomyelitis vaccine
PL...............light perception
  phospholipid
  placebo
  placental lactogen
  Public Law
  pulpolingual
PLA............pulpolinguoaxial
PLa ....pulpolabial
PLD............platelet defect
PLS ....please
  prostaglandin-like substance
PLV.............live poliomyelitis vaccine
  panleukopenia virus
  phenylalanine-lysine-vasopressin
PM ....night
  physical medicine
  polymorphs
  postmortem
  pulpomesial

PMA ....prevalence of gingivitis (papillary, marginal, attached)
progressive muscular atrophy
PMB ....para-hydroxymercuribenzoate
polymorphonuclear basophil
PMD ....primary myocardial disease
progressive muscular dystrophy
PME ....polymorphonuclear eosinophil
PMH ....past medical history
PMI ....point of maximal impulse
point of maximum intensity
PML ....progressive multifocal leukoencephalopathy
PMN ....polymorphonuclear neutrophil
PMP ....past menstrual period
previous menstrual period
PMR ....perinatal mortality rate
physical medicine and rehabilitation
proportionate morbidity ratio
PMS ....phenazine methosulfate
postmitochondrial supernatant
pregnant mare serum
PMSG ....pregnant mare serum gonadotropin
PMT ....Porteus maze test
PN ....perceived noise
percussion note
periarteritis nodosa
peripheral neuropathy
pneumonia
positional nystagmus
Practical Nurse
pyelonephritis
PND ....paroxysmal nocturnal dyspnea
postnasal drainage
postnasal drip
pound
PNH ....paroxysmal nocturnal hemoglobinuria
PNP ....para-nitrophenol
Pediatric Nurse Practitioner
PNPP ....para-nitrophenylphosphate
PNU ....protein nitrogen unit

PO ....by mouth (*per os*) ◀━
parieto-occipital
period of onset
phone order
posterior
postoperative
pO$_2$ ....partial pressure of oxygen
POA............point of application
POB ....phenoxybenzamine
place of birth
Prevention of Blindness
POC............postoperative care
POCUL........cup (*poculum*)
POD ....place of death
postoperative day
PodD ....Doctor of Podiatry
PODx..........preoperative diagnosis
pOH............hydroxyl concentration
POIK ....poikilocyte
POLIO ....poliomyelitis
POLY ....polymorphonuclear leukocyte
POP............plasma oncotic pressure
POS............positive
POS PR ....positive pressure
POSS..........possible
POST..........posterior
postmortem
POSTOP ......postoperative
POT............potassa
potion
PP ....after shaking (*phiala prius agitata*)
near point (*punctum proximum*)
partial pressure
pauperismus
pellagra preventive
permanent partial
pink puffers (emphysema)
pinpoint
postpartum
postprandial
private practice

PP *Continued*

prothrombin-proconvertin
protoporphyrin
proximal phalanx
pulse pressure
pyrophosphate

PPA..............shake well (*phiala prius agitata*)
PPB..............parts per billion
platelet-poor blood
positive-pressure breathing
PPBS...........postprandial blood sugar
PPC..............progressive patient care
PPD..............paraphenylenediamine
purified protein derivative
PPD-S..........Purified Protein Derivative-Standard
ppg..............picopicogram
PPH..............primary pulmonary hypertension
protocollagen proline hydroxylase
postpartum hemorrhage
PPHP..........pseudopseudohypoparathyroidism
PPLO...........pleuropneumonia-like organism
PPM.............parts per million
PPP..............pentose phosphate pathway
PPPI...........primary private practice income
PPR..............Price precipitation reaction
PPS..............postpump syndrome
PPT..............plant protease test
precipitate
prepared
PPV..............positive-pressure ventilation
PQ...............permeability quotient
pyrimethamine-quinine
PR...............far point (*punctum remotum*)
partial remission
peer review
peripheral resistance
pregnancy rate
presbyopia
prism
production rate
professional relations

PR *Continued*

	protein
	public relations
	pulse rate
	through the rectum (*per rectum*)
PRA	plasma renin activity
PRB	Population Reference Bureau
PRBV	placental residual blood volume
PRC	packed red cells
PRCA	pure red cell agenesis
PRD	partial reaction of degeneration
	postradiation dysplasia
PRE	preliminary
PREG	pregnant
PREOP	preoperative
PREP	prepare
PRFM	prolonged rupture of fetal membranes
PRI	phosphoribose isomerase
PRIMIP	woman bearing first child
PRM	phosphoribomutase
	preventive medicine
PRN	as the occasion arises (*pro re nata*)
PRO	prothrombin
PROG	prognosis
PROM	premature rupture of membranes
	prolonged rupture of membranes
PROX	proximal
PRP	pityriasis rubra pilaris
	platelet-rich plasma
	Psychotic Reaction Profile
PRPP	phosphoribosylpyrophosphate
PRT	phosphoribosyltransferase
PRU	peripheral resistance unit
PS	chloropicrin
	per second
	performing scale (IQ)
	periodic syndrome
	physical status
	plastic surgery
	population sample
	Porter-Silber (chromogen)

PS *Continued*

	prescription
	Pseudomonas
	psychiatric
	pulmonary stenosis
	pyloric stenosis
P/S	polyunsaturated to saturated fatty acids ratio
PSA	apply to the affected region
	polyethylene sulfonic acid
PSC	Porter-Silber chromogen
	posterior subcapsular cataract
PSE	portal-systemic encephalopathy
PSG	peak systolic gradient
	presystolic gallop
PSGN	poststreptococcal glomerulonephritis
psi	pounds per square inch
PSP	periodic short pulse
	phenolsulfonphthalein
	positive spike pattern
	progressive supranuclear palsy
PSS	physiological saline solution
	progressive systemic sclerosis
PST	penicillin, streptomycin, and tetracycline
PSW	Psychiatric Social Worker
PSY	psychiatry
	psychology
PSYCH	psychiatry
	psychology
PT	parathyroid
	paroxysmal tachycardia
	patient
	permanent and total
	pharmacy and therapeutics
	physical therapy
	physical training
	pint
	pneumothorax
	prothrombin time
PTA	persistent truncus arteriosus
	phosphotungstic acid
	plasma thromboplastin antecedent
	post-traumatic amnesia

PTA *Continued*

	prior to admission
	prior to arrival
PTAH	phosphotungstic acid hematoxylin
PTB	patellar tendon bearing
	prior to birth
PTC	phenylthiocarbamide
	plasma thromboplastin component
PTD	permanent and total disability
PTE	parathyroid extract
	pulmonary thromboembolism
PTED	pulmonary thromboembolic disease
PTH	parathormone
	parathyroid hormone
	post transfusion hepatitis
PTHS	parathyroid hormone secretion (rate)
PTI	persistent tolerant infection
PTM	post-transfusion mononucleosis
PTMA	phenyltrimethylammonium
PTP	post-tetanic potentiation
	prior to program
PTR	peripheral total resistance
PTS	para-toluenesulfonic acid
PTT	partial thromboplastin time
	particle transport time
PTU	propylthiouracil
PTX	parathyroidectomy
PU	peptic ulcer
	pregnancy urine
PUD	pulmonary disease
PUE	pyrexia of unknown etiology
PUFA	polyunsaturated fatty acid
PUL	pulmonary
PULM	gruel (*pulmentum*)
	pulmonary
PULV	powder (*pulvis*)
PUO	pyrexia of unknown origin
PV	peripheral vascular
	peripheral vein
	peripheral vessels
	plasma volume

PV *Continued*
    polycythemia vera
    portal vein
    postvoiding
    through the vagina (*per vaginam*)
P&V ....pyloroplasty and vagotomy
PVA.............polyvinyl alcohol
PVC.............polyvinyl chloride
    premature ventricular contraction
    pulmonary venous congestion
PVD ....peripheral vascular disease
PVF.............portal venous flow
PVM ....pneumonia virus of mice
PVP.............penicillin V potassium
    peripheral vein plasma
    polyvinylpyrrolidone
    portal venous pressure
PVR.............peripheral vascular resistance
    pulmonary vascular resistance
PVS ....premature ventricular systole
PVT.............paroxysmal ventricular tachycardia
    portal vein thrombosis
    private
PW ....posterior wall
PWB............partial weight-bearing
PWC............physical work capacity
PWI.............posterior wall infarct
PX ....physical examination
    pneumothorax
    prognosis
PXE.............pseudoxanthoma elasticum
PZ ....pancreozymin
PZA.............pyrazinamide
PZ-CCK ....pancreozymin-cholecystokinin
PZI..............protamine zinc insulin

Q

Q ....coulomb
electric quantity
every (*quaque*)
quart
QAM ....every morning
QC ....quinine-colchicine
QCIM ....Quarterly Cumulative Index Medicus
QD ....every day (*quaque die*)
QH ....every hour (*quaque hora*)
Q4H ....every four hours
QID ....four times a day (*quater in die*)
QL ....as much as desired (*quantum libet*)
QM ....every morning (*quaque mane*)
QNS ....quantity not sufficient
QOD ....every other day
qO_2 ....oxygen quotient
QP ....at will (*quantum placeat*)
Qualified Psychiatrist
quanti-Pirquet reaction
QPM ....every night
QQ ....each
QQH ....every four hours (*quaque quarta hora*)
QQHOR ....every hour (*quaque hora*)
QRZ ....wheal reaction time
QS ....enough (*quantum satis*)
QSAD ....to a sufficient quantity
QSUFF ....as much as suffices (*quantum sufficit*)
QT ....quiet
qt ....quart
QUAT ....four
QUICHA ......quantitative inhalation challenge apparatus
QUINT ....fifth
QUOTID ......daily (*quotidie*)
QV ....as much as you like (*quantum vis*)
which see (*quod vide*)

R

R ....Behnken's unit
  organic radical
  radiology
  Rankine (scale)
  Réaumur (scale)
  rectal
  regression coefficient
  remote
  resistance
  respiration
  Rickettsia
  right
  Rinne test
  roentgen
  rough (colony)
  take (*recipe*)
R_A ....airway resistance
R_P ....pulmonary resistance
RA ....renal artery
  rheumatoid arthritis
  right arm
  right atrial
  right atrium
RAB ....Research Advisory Board
RABBI ....Rapid Access Blood Bank Information
RAD ....radial
  radiation absorbed dose
  right axis deviation
  root
RADTS ....rabbit antidog-thymus serum
RAE ....right atrial enlargement
RAF ....rheumatoid arthritis factor
RAH ....right atrial hypertrophy
RAI ....radioactive iodine
RAIU ....radioactive iodine uptake
RAMT ....rabbit antimouse thymocyte
RAO ....right anterior oblique
RAP ....right atrial pressure
RAR ....right arm recumbent
134

RARLS ....rabbit antirat lymphocyte serum
RAS.............renal artery stenosis
             scrapings (*rasurae*)
RAST...........radioallergosorbent test
RATHAS ......rat thymus antiserum
RB...............rating board
RBA ....rose bengal antigen
RBB ....right bundle branch
RBBB..........right bundle branch block
RBC ....red blood cell
             red blood count
RBCM ....red blood cell mass
RBCV..........red blood cell volume
RBE ....relative biological effectiveness
RBF ....renal blood flow
RC...............red cell
             red cell casts
RCA ....right coronary artery
RCBV..........regional cerebral blood volume
RCC ....red cell count
RCD ....relative cardiac dullness
RCF.............red cell folate
             relative centrifugal force
RCM ....red cell mass
             right costal margin
RCR ....respiratory control ratio
RCS.............reticulum cell sarcoma
RCU ....respiratory care unit
RCV ....red cell volume
RD...............Raynaud's disease
             reaction of (to) degeneration
             Registered Dietitian
             resistance determinant
             respiratory disease
             right deltoid
R&D ....Research and Development
rd ....rutherford
RDA ....recommended daily allowance
             recommended dietary allowance
             right dorsoanterior

RDDA..........recommended daily dietary allowance
RDE............receptor destroying enzyme
RDI.............rupture-delivery interval
RDP............right dorsoposterior
RDS.............respiratory distress syndrome
RE...............radium emanation
                regional enteritis
                resting energy
                reticuloendothelial
                right eye
R&E............Research and Education
REC............fresh (*recens*)
RECT..........rectified
RED IN PULV...reduced to powder (*reductus in pulverem*)
REEGT........Registered Electroencephalographic Technician
REF.............renal erythropoietic factor
REF DOC ...referring doctor
REFRAD .....released from active duty
REG ....radioencephalogram
REG UMB ...umbilical region
REHAB ....rehabilitation
REM............rapid eye movement
                removal
                roentgen-equivalent—man
REMP..........roentgen-equivalent—man period
REP.............let it be repeated (*repetatur*)
                roentgen-equivalent—physical
REPT...........let it be repeated
RER ....rough endoplasmic reticulum
RES.............research
                reticuloendothelial system
RESP...........respectively
                respiratory
RETIC ....reticulocyte
RF ....Reitland-Franklin (unit)
                relative fluorescence
                releasing factor
                rheumatic fever
                rheumatoid factor
                root canal, filling of

RFA.............right femoral artery
              right frontoanterior
RFB ....retained foreign body
RFLA ....rheumatoid factor-like activity
RFN ....Registered Fever Nurse
RFP.............right frontoposterior
RFS.............renal function study
RFT.............right frontotransverse
              rod-and-frame test
RFW ....rapid filling wave
RG...............right gluteal
RH...............reactive hyperemia
              relative humidity
              rheumatic
Rh ....Rhesus (factor)
RHBF.........reactive hyperemia blood flow
RHD ....relative hepatic dullness
              rheumatic heart disease
RHEUM.......rheumatic
RHL ....right hepatic lobe
RHLN ....right hilar lymph node
rhm ....roentgen (per) hour (at one) meter
RI................refractive index
              regional ileitis
              respiratory illness
RIA ....radioimmunoassay
RIF..............right iliac fossa
RIFA ....radioiodinated fatty acid
RIHSA.........radioactive iodinated human serum albumin
RISA ....radioiodinated serum albumin
RITC ....rhodamine isothiocyanate
RIU ....radioactive iodine uptake
RK...............rabbit kidney
              right kidney
RKY ....roentgen kymography
RL...............Record Librarian
              right leg
              right lung
R-L..............right to left
R→L............right to left
RLC.............residual lung capacity

RLD ....related living donor
RLF............retrolental fibroplasia
RLL............right lower lobe
RLM ....Regional Library of Medicine
RLN ....recurrent laryngeal nerve
RLP............radiation-leukemia-protection
RLQ............right lower quadrant
RLS ....Ringer's lactate solution
RM ....radical mastectomy
                      respiratory movement
RMA............right mentoanterior
RMK............rhesus monkey kidney
RML ....right middle lobe
RMO ....Regional Medical Officer
                      Resident Medical Officer
RMP ....rapidly miscible pool
                      Regional Medical Program
                      right mentoposterior
RMS ....root-mean-square
RMSF ....Rocky Mountain spotted fever
RMT ....retromolar trigone
                      right mentotransverse
RMV ....respiratory minute volume
RN...............Registered Nurse
RNA ....Registered Nurse Anesthetist
                      ribonucleic acid
RNase..........ribonuclease
RND ....radical neck dissection
RNMS..........Registered Nurse for the Mentally Subnormal
RNP ....ribonucleoprotein
RO...............Ritter-Oleson (technique)
                      rule out
ROA ....right occipitoanterior
ROH ....rat ovarian hyperemia (test)
ROM............range of motion
                      rupture of membranes
ROP............right occipitoposterior
ROS............review of systems
ROT............right occipitotransverse
                      rotating

RP ....reactive protein
                 refractory period
                 Registered Pharmacist
                 rest pain
                 resting pressure
RPA.............right pulmonary artery
RPCF ....Reiter protein complement fixation
RPCFT ....Reiter protein complement fixation test
RPE.............retinal pigment epithelium
RPF.............renal plasma flow
RPG.............retrograde pyelogram
RPGN ....rapidly progressive glomerulonephritis
rpm ....revolutions per minute
RPR.............rapid plasma reagin
RPS.............renal pressor substance
RPV.............right pulmonary veins
RQ...............respiratory quotient
RR...............radiation response
                 Recovery Room
                 renin release
                 respiratory rate
                 response rate
R&R ....rest and recuperation
RR&E..........round, regular, and equal
RR-HPO.......rapid recompression-high pressure oxygen
RRL.............Registered Record Librarian
RRP.............relative refractory period
RRR ....renin-release rate
RS ....Rating Schedule
                 respiratory syncytial
                 right side
RSA.............Rehabilitation Services Administration
                 relative specific activity
                 reticulum cell sarcoma
                 right sacroanterior
RSB.............right sternal border
RSC.............rested-state contraction
RScA ....right scapuloanterior
RSCN ....Registered Sick Children's Nurse
RScP ....right scapuloposterior

RSP ....right sacroposterior
RSR.............regular sinus rhythm
RST ....radiosensitivity test
                right sacrotransverse
RSV.............respiratory syncytial virus
                right subclavian vein
                Rous sarcoma virus
RT ....radiation therapy
                radiotherapy
                radium therapy
                reaction time
                reading test
                recreational therapy
                Registered Technician
                Registered Technologist
                right
                right thigh
                room temperature
RT LAT........right lateral
RTA.............renal tubular acidosis
RTD.............retarded
                routine test dilution
RTF ....replication and transfer
                resistance transfer factor
                respiratory tract fluid
RTN.............return
RU...............rat unit
                resistance unit
                right upper
RUB ....red (*ruber*)
RUL ....right upper lobe
RUQ ....right upper quadrant
RUR ....resin-uptake ratio
RURTI.........recurrent upper respiratory tract infection
RV...............rat virus
                residual volume
                respiratory volume
                right ventricle
                rubella virus
RVB ....red venous blood

RVD ....relative vertebral density
RVE ....right ventricular enlargement
RVEDP........right ventricular end-diastolic pressure
RVH ....right ventricular hypertrophy
RVI ....relative value index
RVP............red veterinary petrolatum
RVR ....renal vascular resistance
               resistance to venous return
RVRA ....renal vein renin activity
               renal venous renin assay
RVRC ....renal vein renin concentration
RVS............Relative Value Study (Schedule)
RVT............renal vein thrombosis
RW ....ragweed
RX...............take (*recipe*)
               treatment

S

S ....half (*semis*)
label (*signa*)
left (*sinister*)
sacral
Salmonella
Schistosoma
second
single
smooth
soluble
spherical lens
Spirillum
Staphylococcus
Streptococcus
subject
supravergence
surgery
Svedberg unit of sedimentation coefficient
without (*sine*)
write (*signa*)
S OP S.........if it is necessary (*si opus sit*)
S ROMANUM...sigmoid colon
SA ....according to art (*secundum artem*)
salicylic acid
sarcoma
secondary amenorrhea
secondary anemia
sensation unit
serum albumin
sinoatrial
slightly active
specific activity
Stokes-Adams
surface area
sustained action
sympathetic activity
SAB..............significant asymptomatic bacteriuria
SACD ....subacute combined degeneration
SAD..............source to axis distance

142

SAG.............Swiss agammaglobulinemia
SAH.............subarachnoid hemorrhage
SAI.............Social Adequacy Index
SAL.............according to the rules of art (*secundum artis leges*)
             saline
SAM ....sulfated acid mucopolysaccharide
SAMA.........Student American Medical Association
SAP ....serum alkaline phosphatase
             systemic arterial pressure
SAS ....supravalvular aortic stenosis
SAT ....saturated
             Scholastic Aptitude Test
SB ....serum bilirubin
             single breath
             Stanford-Binet (test)
             sternal border
             stillbirth
SBE.............subacute bacterial endocarditis
SBF.............splanchnic blood flow
SBH ....State Board of Health
SBP.............systemic blood pressure
             systolic blood pressure
SBS............social-breakdown syndrome
SBT............single-breath test
SBTI...........soy-bean trypsin inhibitor
SC ....closure of the semilunar valves
             sacrococcygeal
             Self-Care
             semicircular
             semiclosed
             service connected
             sick call
             sickle cell
             single chemical
             Special Care
             sternoclavicular
             subcutaneous
             succinylcholine
             sugar-coated
SCAT...........a box (*scatula*)
             sheep cell agglutination test

SCC.............Services for Crippled Children
                squamous cell carcinoma
SCD.............service-connected disability
ScD ....Doctor of Science
ScDA ....scapulodextra anterior
ScDP ....scapulodextra posterior
SCH.............succinylcholine
SCHED........schedule
SCHIZ ....schizophrenia
SCI.............structured clinical interview
SCK.............serum creatine kinase
ScLA ....scapulolaeva anterior
ScLP...........scapulolaeva posterior
SCM ....State Certified Midwife
SCOP...........scopolamine
SCP.............single-celled protein
SCPK ....serum creatine phosphokinase
SCR.............scruple
SCT.............sex chromatin test
                staphylococcal clumping test
SCUBA........self-contained underwater breathing apparatus
SD...............septal defect
                serum defect
                skin dose
                spontaneous delivery
                standard deviation
                streptodornase
                sudden death
S/D.............systolic to diastolic
SDA.............sacrodextra anterior
                specific dynamic action
SDCL ....symptom distress check list
SDH ....serine dehydrase
                sorbitol dehydrogenase
                succinate dehydrogenase
SDM ....standard deviation of the mean
SDO.............sudden-dosage onset
SDP.............sacrodextra posterior
SDS.............Self-Rating Depression Scale
                sensory deprivation syndrome
                sodium dodecyl sulfate

SDS *Continued*

        sudden death syndrome

SDT............sacrodextra transversa

SDU ....Standard Deviation Unit

SE ....himself

        standard error

        Starr-Edwards (prosthesis)

sec...............second

SED............skin erythema dose

        spondyloepiphyseal dysplasia

        stool (*sedes*)

SEE............standard error of the estimate

SEG............segmented (leukocyte)

        sonoencephalogram

SEM ....scanning electron microscopy

        standard error of the mean

SEMI...........half

SEMID ....half a drachm

SEMIH ....half an hour

SEP.............sensory evoked potential

        systolic ejection period

SEQ.............sequela

        sequestrum

SEQ LUCE...the next day (*sequenti luce*)

SER.............smooth endoplasmic reticulum

        systolic ejection rate

SERV ....keep (*serva*)

        preserve

SES ....socioeconomic status

SET.............systolic ejection time

SEV.............severe

        severed

SF ....scarlet fever

        shell fragment

        shrapnel fragment

        spinal fluid

Sf ....Svedberg flotation units

SFD............short food drape

SFF ....specific-pathogen free

SFP ....screen filtration pressure

        spinal fluid pressure

SFS ....split function study
SFT ....skinfold thickness
SFW ....shell fragment wound
　　　　　　　shrapnel fragment wound
SG ....serum globulin
　　　　　　　signs
　　　　　　　skin graft
　　　　　　　specific gravity
S-G ....Sachs-Georgi (test)
SGA.............small for gestational age
SGO.............Surgeon-General's Office
　　　　　　　Surgery, Gynecology, and Obstetrics
SGOT...........serum glutamic oxalic transaminase
　　　　　　　serum glutamic oxaloacetic transaminase
SGP ....serine glycerophosphatide
SGPT...........serum glutamic pyruvic transaminase
SGV.............salivary gland virus
SH...............serum hepatitis
　　　　　　　sex hormone
　　　　　　　sinus histiocytosis
　　　　　　　shoulder
　　　　　　　social history
　　　　　　　State Hospital
　　　　　　　Student Health
　　　　　　　sulfhydryl
　　　　　　　surgical history
SHB ....sulfhemoglobin
SHBD..........serum hydroxybutyrate dehydrogenase
SHES...........School Health Education Study
SHG.............synthetic human gastrin
SHO.............secondary hypertrophic osteoarthropathy
　　　　　　　Student Health Organization
SI ....sacro-iliac
　　　　　　　saturation index
　　　　　　　self-inflicted
　　　　　　　seriously ill
　　　　　　　serum iron
　　　　　　　soluble insulin
　　　　　　　stroke index
SI NON VAL...if it is not enough (*si non valeat*)
SI OP SIT.....if it is necessary (*si opus sit*)

SI VIR PERM...if the strength will permit (*si vires permittant*)
SIADH.........syndrome of inappropriate antidiuretic hormone
SICD ....serum isocitric dehydrogenase
SID..............sudden infant death
SIDS............sudden infant death syndrome
SIECUS.......Sex Information and Education Council of the
United States
SIG..............let it be labeled (*signetur*)
significant
SIG N PRO...label with the proper name (*signa nomine proprio*)
SIJ..............sacro-iliac joint
SIMUL.........at the same time
SING ....of each
SISI.............short-increment sensitivity index
SIW ....self-inflicted wound
SJR ....Shinawora-Jones-Reinhart (units)
SK...............Sloan-Kettering
streptokinase
SKSD ....streptokinase-streptodornase
SL ....according to law (*secundum legem*)
sensation level
slight
streptolysin
SLA.............sacrolaeva anterior
SLD.............serum lactic dehydrogenase
SLDH ....serum lactic dehydrogenase
SLE ....St. Louis encephalitis
systemic lupus erythematosus
SLEV...........St. Louis encephalitis virus
SLI..............splenic localization index
SLKC ....superior limbic keratoconjunctivitis
SLN.............superior laryngeal nerve
SLO.............streptolysin-*O*
SLP ....sacrolaeva posterior
SLR.............straight leg raising
Streptococcus lactis R
SLT ....sacrolaeva transversa
SM...............simple mastectomy
skim milk
small
streptomycin

SM *Continued*
        submucous
        suction method
        systolic mean
        systolic murmur
        symptoms
SMA ....Sequential Multiple Analysis
        superior mesenteric artery
SMC ....special monthly compensation
        State Medical Society
SMI ....Senior Medical Investigator
SMJAB ....State Medical Journal Advertising Bureau
SMO ....Medical Officer of Schools
        Senior Medical Officer
        slip made out
SMON..........subacute myelo-optical neuropathy
SMP ....slow-moving protease
        special monthly pension
SMR ....somnolent metabolic rate
        standard mortality ratio
        standardized mortality ratio
        submucous resection
SMSA ....Standard Metropolitan Statistical Area
SN...............according to nature (*secundum naturam*)
        serum-neutralizing
        Standard Nomenclature
        Student Nurse
        suprasternal notch
SNAI ....Standard Nomenclature of Athletic Injuries
SNB ....scalene node biopsy
SNDO ....Standard Nomenclature of Diseases and Operations
SNOP ....Systematized Nomenclature of Pathology
SNS.............Society of Neurological Surgeons
SO ....salpingo-oophorectomy
SOB............short of breath
SOC............sequential-type oral contraceptive
SOL............solution
        space-occupying lesion
SOLN ....solution
SOLV...........dissolve (*solve*)

SOM ....secretory otitis media
                serous otitis media
                sulformethoxine
SOMOS ....Society of Military Orthopedic Surgeons
SOP ....standing operative procedure
SOS ....if it is necessary (*si opus sit*)
SOTT ....synthetic medium old tuberculin trichloracetic acid
                precipitated
SP ....shunt procedure
                skin potential
                species
                spirit (*spiritus*)
                steady potential
                summating potential
                suprapubic
                symphysis pubis
                systolic pressure
SP GR..........specific gravity
SPA ....suprapubic aspiration
SPAI............steroid protein activity index
SPBI ....serum protein-bound iodine
SPCA...........serum prothrombin-conversion accelerator
SPCK ....serum creatine phosphokinase
SPEC...........specimen
SPF ....specific-pathogen free
                split products of fibrin
SPH.............secondary pulmonary hemosiderosis
                spherical
                spherical lens
SPI..............serum precipitable iodine
SPIR............spirit (*spiritus*)
SPL ....sound pressure level
                spontaneous lesion
SPN.............Student Practical Nurse
SPONT ....spontaneous (delivery)
SPP ....suprapubic prostatectomy
SPT ....spirit
SQ ....social quotient
                square
                subcutaneous

SR ....sarcoplasmic reticulum
secretion rate
sedimentation rate
sensitization response
service record
sigma reaction
sinus rhythm
skin resistance
superior rectus
system review
systemic resistance
systems research
SRBC ....sheep red blood cells
SRC.............sedimented red cells
sheep red cells
SRF ....somatotropin-releasing factor
split renal function
SRFS...........split renal function study
SRM ....Standard Reference Material
SRN.............Student Registered Nurse
SRNA ....soluble ribonucleic acid
SRR.............slow rotation room
SRS ....slow-reacting substance
Social and Rehabilitation Service
SRSA...........slow-reacting substance of anaphylaxis
SRT ....speech reception test
speech reception threshold
Stroke Rehabilitation Technician
SS ....saturated solution
side to side
signs and symptoms
soapsuds
statistically significant
subaortic stenosis
sum of squares
supersaturated
ss ....one-half (*semissen*)
SSA ....salicylsalicylic acid
skin-sensitizing antibody
Social Security Administration
sulfosalicylic acid (test)

SSD ....source to skin distance
              sum of square deviations
SSE ....soapsuds enema
SSKI...........saturated solution of potassium iodide
SSN............severely subnormal
SSP ....Sanarelli-Shwartzman phenomenon
              subacute sclerosing panencephalitis
SSPE ....subacute sclerosing panencephalitis
SSS ....layer upon layer (*stratum super stratum*)
              specific soluble substance
SSU ....sterile supply unit
SSV ....under a poison label (*sub signo veneni*)
ST ....let it stand (*stet*)
              sternothyroid
              straight
              subtalar
              subtotal
              surface tension
STA ....serum thrombotic accelerator
STAB...........stabnuclear neutrophil
STAPH ....staphylococcus
STAT ....immediately (*statim*) — *first dose*
stat ....German unit of radium emanation
STC ....soft tissue calcification
STD ....saturated
              skin test dose
              skin to tumor distance
STET ....let it stand
STH ....somatotropic hormone
STK ....streptokinase
STM............streptomycin
STP ....scientifically treated petroleum
              standard temperature and pressure
STPD...........standard temperature and pressure, dry (0° C.,
              760 mm. Hg)
STR ....streptococcus
STREP.........streptococcus
STS ....serologic test for syphilis
              standard test for syphilis
STSG ....split thickness skin graft
STT ....serial thrombin time

STU..............skin test unit
STVA...........subtotal villose atrophy
STYCAR......Screening Tests for Young Children and Retardates
SU...............let him take (*sumat*)
SUA.............serum uric acid
                single umbilical artery
SUBCU........subcutaneous
SUBQ..........subcutaneous
SUD ....sudden unexpected death
                sudden unexplained death
SUID...........sudden unexplained infant death
SUM............let him take (*sumat*)
SUN ....serum urea nitrogen
SUP.............superficial
                superior
SURG ....surgery
SUS.............stained urinary sediment
SUUD..........sudden unexpected unexplained death
SV ....alcoholic spirit (*spiritus vini*)
                severe
                simian virus
                snake venom
                stroke volume
                subclavian vein
                supravital
SVAS...........supravalvular aortic stenosis
SVC.............slow vital capacity
                superior vena cava
SVCG ....spatial vectorcardiogram
SVD.............spontaneous vaginal delivery
                spontaneous vertex delivery
SVI..............stroke volume index
SVM ....syncytiovascular membrane
SVR.............rectified spirit of wine (*spiritus vini rectificatus*)
                systemic vascular resistance
SVT ....proof spirit (*spiritus vini tenuis*)
SW ....Social Worker
                spiral wound
                stroke work

SWI ....stroke work index
SX ....signs
              symptoms
SYM ....symmetrical
              symptoms
SYMP ....symptoms
SYR.............syrup
SZ ....schizophrenia

T

T	Taenia
	temperature
	tension, intraocular
	thoracic
	time
	Treponema
	Trichophyton
	Trypanosoma
	tumor
t	temporal
	ter- (three times)
	tertiary
	test of significance
T+	increased tension
T−	decreased tension
T$_{1/2}$	half-life
T$_3$	triiodothyronine
T$_4$	thyroxine, levothyroxine, tetraiodothyronine
TA	alkaline tuberculin
	therapeutic abortion
	titratable acid
	toxin-antitoxin
TAB	tablet
	typhoid, paratyphoid A, and paratyphoid B
TACE	tripara-anisylchloroethylene
TAD	thoracic asphyxiant dystrophy
TAF	albumose-free tuberculin
	toxoid-antitoxin floccules
	trypsin-aldehyde-fuchsin
TAH	total abdominal hysterectomy
TAL	of such (*talis*)
	thymic alymphoplasia
TAM	toxoid-antitoxin mixture
TAME	toluene-sulpho-trypsin arginine methyl ester
TAO	thromboangiitis obliterans
	triacetyloleandomycin
TAPVD	total anomalous pulmonary venous drainage
TAR	thrombocytopenia with absence of the radius

TAT ....tetanus antitoxin
               thematic apperception test
               thromboplastin activation test
               total antitryptic activity
               toxin-antitoxin
               tyrosine aminotransferase
TB ....toluidine blue
               total base
               total body
               tracheobronchitis
               tubercle bacillus
               tuberculosis
TBA.............tertiary butylacetate
               testosterone-binding affinity
               thiobarbituric acid
TBC.............tuberculosis
TBD ....total body density
TBF.............total body fat
TBG.............thyroxine-binding globulin
TBGP ....total blood granulocyte pool
TBI.............thyroid-binding index
               total body irradiation
TBK ....total body potassium
TBM ....tuberculous meningitis
TBN ....bacillus emulsion
TBP.............thyroxine-binding protein
TBPA ....thyroxine-binding prealbumin
TB-RD ....tuberculosis-respiratory disease
TBS ....total body solute
               tribromosalicylanilide
               triethanolamine-buffered saline
tbsp ....tablespoonful
TBT.............tolbutamide test
               tracheobronchial toilet
TBV.............total blood volume
TBW ....total body water
               total body weight
TBX.............whole body irradiation
TC ....taurocholate
               temperature compensation

TC *Continued*

        tetracycline
        tissue culture
        to contain
        total capacity
        total cholesterol
        tubocurarine

TCA............tricarboxylic acid
        trichloroacetate
        trichloroacetic acid

TCAP...........trimethylcetylammonium pentachlorophenate
TCC............trichlorocarbanilide
TCD............tissue culture dose
TCD$_{50}$...........median tissue culture dose
TCE............trichloroethylene
TCF............total coronary flow
TCH............total circulating hemoglobin
TCI............to come in
        transient cerebral ischemia

TCID...........tissue culture infective dose
TCID$_{50}$.........median tissue culture infective dose
TCIE...........transient cerebral ischemic episode
TCM............tissue culture medium
TCP............therapeutic continuous penicillin
TCSA...........tetrachlorosalicylanilide
TCT............thrombin clotting time
        thyrocalcitonin

TD...............tetanus-diptheria
        therapy discontinued
        thoracic duct
        three times a day
        threshold of discomfort
        thymus-dependent
        time disintegration
        to deliver
        tone decay
        torsion dystonia
        total disability
        transverse diameter
        treatment discontinued

TDF.............thoracic duct fistula
                thoracic duct flow
TDI.............toluene-diisocyanate
                total-dose infusion
TDL.............thoracic duct lymph
TDP.............thoracic duct pressure
                thymidine diphosphate
TDS.............three dimes a day (*ter die sumendum*)
TDT.............tone decay test
TE ....tetanus
                threshold energy
                tissue-equivalent
                tooth extracted
                total estrogen (excretion)
                tracheo-esophageal
TEA.............tetraethylammonium
TEAC ....tetraethylammonium chloride
TEE.............tyrosine ethyl ester
TEEP...........tetraethyl pyrophosphate
TEF.............tracheo-esophageal fistula
TEIB ....triethyleneiminobenzoquinone
TEL.............tetraethyl lead
TEM ....transmission electron microscopy
                triethylenemelamine
TEN.............toxic epidermal necrolysis
TENAC........tenaculum
TEP.............thromboendophlebectomy
TEPP...........tetraethyl pyrophosphate
TER.............three times
                threefold
TES ....trismethylaminoethanesulfonic acid
TET ....tetralogy of Fallot
TETD...........tetraethylthiuram-disulfide
TF ....tactile fremitus
                tetralogy of Fallot
                thymol flocculation
                tissue-damaging factor
                to follow
                total flow
                transfer factor

TF *Continued*
> tuberculin filtrate
> tubular fluid

TFA..............total fatty acids
TFE..............tetrafluoroethylene
TFS ....testicular feminization syndrome
TG ....thioguanine
> thyroglobulin
> toxic goiter
> triglyceride

TGA..............transposition of the great arteries
TGAR ....total graft area rejected
TGFA...........triglyceride fatty acid
TGL..............triglyceride
> triglyceride lipase

TGT..............thromboplastin generation test
> thromboplastin generation time

TGV..............thoracic gas volume
> transposition of the great vessels

TH...............thoracic
> thyrohyoid

THA..............total hydroxyapatite
THAM..........trihydroxymethylaminomethane
THC..............tetrahydrocannabinol
THDOC........tetrahydrodeoxycorticosterone
THE..............tetrahydrocortisone
THER ....therapy
THF..............humoral thymic factor
> tetrahydrocortisol
> tetrahydrofolic acid

THFA ....tetrahydrofolic acid
THO..............tritiated water
THP..............total hydroxyproline
TI ....thoracic index
> time interval
> tricuspid incompetence
> tricuspid insufficiency

TIA..............transient ischemic attack
TIBC ....total iron-binding capacity
TIC..............trypsin-inhibitory capacity

TID.............three times a day (*ter in die*)
            titrated initial dose
TIE.............transient ischemic episode
TIN.............three times a night (*ter in nocte*)
TINCT ....tincture
TIS ....tumor in situ
TIVC ....thoracic inferior vena cava
TKA............transketolase activity
TKD ....tokodynamometer
TKG............tokodynagraph
TL ....Team Leader
            time lapse
            time-limited
            total lipids
            tubal ligation
TLC............tender loving care
            thin-layer chromatography
            total L-chain concentration
            total lung capacity
            total lung compliance
TLD............thermoluminescent dosimeter
T/LD$_{100}$.........minimum dose causing death or malformation of
            100 per cent of fetuses
TLE............thin-layer electrophoresis
TLQ............total living quotient
TLV............threshold limit value
TM.............temporomandibular
            trademark
            transmetatarsal
            tympanic membrane
Tm..............maximal tubular excretory capacity of the kidneys
TMAS ....Taylor Manifest Anxiety Scale
TmG ....maximal tubular reabsorption of glucose
TMJ............temporomandibular joint
TML ....tetramethyl lead
TMP ....thymidine monophosphate
            trimethoprim
TMTD ....tetramethylthiuram disulfide
TMV ....tobacco mosaic virus
TN..............total negatives
            true-negative

Tn...............normal intraocular tension
TNAS..........Tuberculosis Nursing Advisory Service
TND ....term normal delivery
TNI.............total nodal irradiation
TNM ....(primary) tumor, (regional lymph) nodes, (remote) metastases (system)
TNT............trinitrotoluene
TNTC..........too numerous to count
TO ....original tuberculin
                   telephone order
                   tincture of opium
TOA............tubo-ovarian abscess
TOCP..........triorthocresyl phosphate
TONOC.......tonight
TOPS..........Take Off Pounds Sensibly
TOPV..........trivalent oral poliovirus vaccine
TOT PROT ...total protein
TP ....temperature and pressure
                   thrombocytopenic purpura
                   total positives
                   total protein
                   true-positive
                   tryptophan
                   tube precipitin
                   tuberculin precipitation
TPA............Treponema pallidum agglutination
TPBF..........total pulmonary blood flow
TPCF..........Treponema pallidum complement fixation
TPG............transplacental gradient
TPH............transplacental hemorrhage
TPI.............Treponema pallidium immobilization
                   triose phosphate isomerase
TPIA...........Treponema pallidum immobilization (immune) ad-herence
TPM ....triphenylmethane
TPN............triphosphopyridine nucleotide
TPNH ....reduced triphosphopyridine nucleotide
TPP............thiamine pyrophosphate
TPR............temperature, pulse, and respiration
                   testosterone production rate
                   total peripheral resistance

TPR *Continued*

total pulmonary resistance
TPS ....tumor polysaccharide substance
TPT ....typhoid-paratyphoid (vaccine)
TPTZ ....tripyridyltriazine
TPVR...........total pulmonary vascular resistance
TQ ....tourniquet
TR ....tetrazolium reduction
therapeutic radiology
time released
tincture
total resistance
total response
trace
tuberculin R (new tuberculin)
TRA.............transaldolase
TRAM..........Treatment Rating Assessment Matrix
Treatment Response Assessment Method
TRBF ....total renal blood flow
TRC.............tanned red cell
total ridge-count
TRF ....thyrotropin-releasing factor
TRH.............thyrotropin-releasing hormone
TRI.............tetrazolium-reduction inhibition
TRIC ....trachoma-inclusion conjunctivitis
TRIT...........triturate
TRK.............transketolase
TRMC..........tetramethylrhodamino-isothiocyanate
TROCH........trochiscus
TRP ....tubular reabsorption of phosphate
TRPT...........theoretical renal phosphorus threshold
TRU.............turbidity-reducing unit
TS ....test solution
thoracic surgery
total solids
Training School
triple strength
tropical sprue
TSA ....technical surgical assistance
trypticase soy agar
T₄SA ....thyroxine-specific activity

TSB ....trypticase soy broth
TSC ....thiosemicarbizide
TSD ....target skin distance
　　　　　　　Tay-Sachs disease
　　　　　　　theory of signal detectability
TSE ....trisodium edetate
TSF ....tissue coding factor
TSH ....thyroid-stimulating hormone
TSI ....triple sugar iron (agar)
TSP ....total serum protein
tsp ....teaspoonful
TSPAP ....total serum prostatic acid phosphatase
TSR ....thyroid to serum ratio
TSS ....tropical splenomegaly syndrome
TST ....tumor skin test
TSTA ....tumor-specific transplantation antigen
TSY ....trypticase soy yeast
TT ....tetrazol
　　　　　　　thrombin time
　　　　　　　thymol turbidity
　　　　　　　tooth, treatment of
　　　　　　　total thyroxine
　　　　　　　total time
　　　　　　　transit time
　　　　　　　transthoracic
TTC ....triphenyltetrazolium chloride
TTH ....thyrotropic hormone
　　　　　　　tritiated thymidine
TTI ....time-tension index (tension time index)
TTP ....thrombotic thrombocytopenic purpura
　　　　　　　thymidine triphosphate
TTS ....temporary threshold shift
TTT ....tolbutamide tolerance test
TU ....thiouracil
　　　　　　　toxic unit
　　　　　　　tuberculin unit
TUBERC .....tuberculosis
TUG ....total urinary gonadotropin
TUR ....transurethral resection
TURB ....transurethral resection of the bladder
TURP ....transurethral resection of the prostate

TUS.............cough (*tussis*)
TV ....tidal volume
              trial visit
              tuberculin volutin
TVC............timed vital capacity
              total volume capacity
              transvaginal cone
TVH............total vaginal hysterectomy
TW ....tap water
TWL ....transepidermal water loss
TX..............traction
              treatment
TY ....type
              typhoid
TZ ....tuberculin zymoplastic

U

U	unit
	unknown
	upper
	urology
UA	umbilical artery
	unaggregated
	uric acid
	urine analysis
	uterine aspiration
UB	ultimobranchial body
UBBC	unsaturated vitamin B_{12}-binding capacity
UBF	uterine blood flow
UBI	ultraviolet blood irradiation
UC	ulcerative colitis
	ultracentrifugal
	unchanged
	unclassifiable
	unit clerk
	urea clearance
	urethral catheterization
U&C	usual and customary
UCD	usual childhood diseases
UCG	urinary chorionic gonadotropin
UCHD	usual childhood diseases
UCO	urethral catheter out
UCP	urinary coproporphyrin
UCS	unconditioned stimulus
	unconscious
UD	urethral discharge
	uroporphyrinogen decarboxylase
UDP	uridine diphosphate
UDPG	uridine diphosphoglucose
UDPGA	uridine diphosphoglucuronic acid
UDPGT	uridine diphosphoglucuronyl transferase
UE	upper extremity
UFA	unesterified fatty acid
UG	urogenital
UGI	upper gastrointestinal
UH	upper half

UI................uroporphyrin isomerase
UIBC...........unsaturated iron-binding capacity
UIF ....undegraded insulin factor
UIQ ....upper inner quadrant
UK ....unknown
                urokinase
UL...............upper lobe
U&L ....upper and lower
ULQ ....upper left quadrant
UM ....uracil mustard
UMB............umbilicus
UMP............uridine monophosphate
UN...............urea nitrogen
UNG............ointment (*unguentum*)
uni-..............one
UNK............unknown
UNKN ....unknown
UOQ ....upper outer quadrant
UP...............upright posture
                ureteropelvic
                uroporphyrin
U/P..............urine-plasma ratio
UPG ....uroporphyrinogen
UPI ....uteroplacental insufficiency
UPJ ....ureteropelvic junction
UPOR ....usual place of residence
UR...............upper respiratory
                urine
                utilization review
URD ....upper respiratory disease
URI ....upper respiratory infection
URQ ....upper right quadrant
URTI ....upper respiratory tract infection
US ....ultrasonic
USAN ....United States Adopted Name
USASI ....United States of America Standards Institute
USD ....United States Dispensatory
USDA ....United States Department of Agriculture
USMH.........United States Marine Hospital
USN ....ultrasonic nebulizer

USO............unilateral salpingo-oophorectomy
USP.............United States Pharmacopeia
USPHS ....United States Public Health Service
USR.............unheated serum reagin (test)
USVB..........United States Veterans Bureau
UT DICT.....as directed (*ut dictum*)
UTBG..........unbound thyroxine-binding globulin
UTEND........to be used (*utendus*)
UTI..............urinary tract infection
UTP.............uridine triphosphate
UU ....urine urobilinogen
UV..............ultraviolet
                umbilical vein
                urinary volume

V

V	see (*vide*)
	vein
	Vibrio
	vision
	visual acuity
	voice
	volume
V$_T$	tidal volume
v	very
	volt
VA	vacuum aspiration
	ventriculoatrial
	vertebral artery
	Veterans Administration
	visual acuity
Va	alveolar ventilation
	visual acuity
VAG	vagina
	vaginal
VAG HYST ...	vaginal hysterectomy
VAH	Veterans Administration Hospital
VALE	visual acuity, left eye
VAMP	vincristine, amethopterin, 6-mercaptopurine, and prednisone
VAR	variation
VARE	visual acuity, right eye
VASC	vascular
	Verbal Auditory Screen for Children
VB	viable birth
	vinblastine
VBS	veronal-buffered saline
VBS:FBS	veronal-buffered saline–fetal bovine serum
VC	acuity of color vision
	vena cava
	ventilatory capacity
	vincristine
	vital capacity
VCG	vectorcardiogram
VCR	vincristine

VD...............vapor density
            venereal disease
VDA ....visual discriminatory acuity
VDBR..........volume of distribution of bilirubin
VDEL ....Venereal Disease Experimental Laboratory
VDG ....venereal disease — gonorrhea
            voiding
VDH ....valvular disease of the heart
VDL ....visual detection level
VDM............vasodepressor material
VDP ....vincristine, daunorubicin, prednisone
VDRL ....Venereal Disease Research Laboratories
VDRS ....Verdun Depression Rating Scale
VDS............venereal disease — syphilis
VE...............volumic ejection
V&E ....Vinethene and ether
VEE ....Venezuelan equine encephalomyelitis
VEM............vasoexcitor material
VENT ....ventricular
VEP............visual evoked potential
VER ....visual evoked response
VES............bladder
            vesicular
VESIC ....blister (*vesicula*)
VF...............left leg (electrode)
            ventricular fibrillation
            ventricular fluid
            visual field
            vocal fremitus
VFP............ventricular fluid pressure
VG...............ventricular gallop
VH...............vaginal hysterectomy
            venous hematocrit
            viral hepatitis
VHD ....viral hematodepressive disease
VHF ....visual half-field
VI................volume index
VIA ....virus-inactivating agent
VIB ....vibration
VIG ....vaccinia-immune globulin
VIN ....wine (*vinum*)
VIP..............very important patient

VIS..............vaginal irrigation smear
VIT..............vitamin
yolk (*vitellus*)
VIT CAP......vital capacity
VL...............left arm (electrode)
VLB............vinblastine
VLDL..........very low-density lipoprotein
VLDLP........very low density lipoprotein
VM..............viomycin
voltmeter
VMA...........vanillylmandelic acid
VN...............virus neutralizing
Visiting Nurse
Vocational Nurse
VNA............Visiting Nurse Association
VO...............verbal order
VOD............vision, right eye
VOL..............volume
VOS.............dissolved in yolk of egg (*vitello ovi solutus*)
vision, left eye
VP...............vasopressin
venipuncture
venous pressure
Voges-Proskauer (reaction)
volume-pressure
vulnerable period
V&P............vagotomy and pyloroplasty
VPB............ventricular premature beat
VPC.............ventricular premature contraction
volume per cent
VPRC..........volume of packed red cells
V/Q.............ventilation-perfusion
VR...............right arm (electrode)
valve replacement
vascular resistance
venous return
ventilation ratio
vocal resonance
vocational rehabilitation
VRA............Vocational Rehabilitation Administration
VRBC..........red blood cell volume

VR&E..........vocational rehabilitation and education
VRI ....viral respiratory infection
VRP.............very reliable product (written on prescription)
VS ....against
vaccination scar
venisection
verbal scale (IQ)
vital signs
voids
volumetric solution
without glasses
vs ....vibration seconds
VsB ....bleeding in the arm (*venaesectio brachii*)
VSD.............ventricular septal defect
VSOK ....vital signs normal
VSS ....vital signs stable
VSULA ....vaccination scar upper left arm
VSV.............vesicular stomatitis virus
VSW ....ventricular stroke work
VT ....tidal volume
vacuum tuberculin
ventricular tachycardia
V&T.............volume and tension
VTSRS.........Verdun Target Symptom Rating Scale
VV...............veins
viper venom
v/v ....volume for volume
V/VI ....grade 5 on a 6 grade basis
VW ....vessel wall
von Willebrand's disease
VZ ....varicella-zoster

W

W	water
	Weber (test)
	week
	wehnelt (unit of hardness roentgen rays)
	weight
	widowed
	wife
	with
W+	weakly positive
w	watt
WA	Woman's Auxiliary
WAIS	Wechsler's Adult Intelligence Scale
WASAMA	Woman's Auxiliary to the Student American Medical Association
WB	weight bearing
	Willowbrook (virus)
	whole blood
	whole body
WBC	white blood cell
	white blood count
WBF	whole-blood folate
WBH	whole-blood hematocrit
WBR	whole body radiation
WC	ward clerk
	water closet
	white cell
	white cell casts
	whooping cough
	work capacity
WC'	whole complement
WCC	white cell count
WD	wallerian degeneration
	well-developed
	well-differentiated
	with disease
WDWN	well-developed, well-nourished
WE	Western encephalitis
	Western encephalomyelitis
WEE	Western equine encephalomyelitis

WF ....Weil-Felix (reaction)
               white female
WFR............Weil-Felix reaction
WG ....water gauge
WH..............well-healed
WHO............World Health Organization
WHOIRP......World Health Organization International Reference
               Preparation
WIA.............wounded in action
WISC...........Wechsler's Intelligence Scale for Children
WK..............weak
               week
               Wernicke-Korsakoff (syndrome)
WL ....waiting list
               wavelength
               work load
WM..............white male
               whole milk
WMA ....World Medical Association
WMF ....white middle-aged female
WMM..........white middle-aged male
WMR ....work metabolic rate
WN..............well-nourished
WNF............well-nourished female
WNL............within normal limits
WNM ....well-nourished male
WO ....without
W/O ....water in oil
WP ....weakly positive
               working point
WPRS ....Wittenborn Psychiatric Rating Scale
WPW ....Wolff-Parkinson-White (syndrome)
WR ....Wassermann reaction
               weakly reactive
               wrist
WRC............washed red cells
WRE............whole ragweed extract
WS ....water swallow
wx ....watts second

WSMSA .... Washington Standard Metropolitan Statistical Area
WT .... weight
                white
WV .... whispered voice
w/v .... weight per volume

X

X ....homeopathic symbol for the decimal scale of
                potencies
                Kienböck's unit of x-ray dosage
                magnification
                removal of
                respirations (anesthesia chart)
                start of anesthesia
                times
XDP ....xeroderma pigmentosum
XM ....crossmatch
XP ....xeroderma pigmentosum
XR ....x-ray
XRT ....X-ray Technician
XS ....excess
                xiphisternum

Y

Y ....year
yd ....yard
YF ....yellow fever
YO ....year old
YOB ....year of birth
yr ....year
YS ....yellow spot (of the retina)
yolk sac

Z

Z ....zero
................Zuckung (contraction)
z ....atomic number
Z/D ....zero defects
ZE ....Zollinger-Ellison (syndrome)
Z/G ....zoster immune globulin
ZIG ....zoster immune globulin
Zz ....ginger
Z, Z′, Z″ ....increasing degrees of contraction

Symbols

Symbol	Meaning	Symbol	Meaning
Ⓛ	left	$\bar{a}$	before
Ⓜ	murmur	$\bar{c}$	with
Ⓡ	right trademark	$\bar{s}$	without
⊙	start of operation	?	question of questionable possible
⊗	end of operation	~	approximate
□	male	±	not definite
○	female	↓	decreased depression
♂	male	↑	elevation increased
♀	female	⇧	up
*	birth	→	causes transfer to
†	death	←	is due to
τ	life (time)	⊖	normal
τ¹/₂	half-life (time)		
$\bar{p}$	after		

$\sqrt{c}$	check with	°	degree
φ	none	′	foot
$\vee$	systolic blood pressure	″	inch
$\wedge$	diastolic blood pressure	$\ddot{\text{ii}}$	two
#	gauge number weight	/	of per
24°	24 hours	:	ratio (is to)
Δt	time interval	+	positive present
3 = D	delayed double diffusion (test)	−	absent negative
606	arsphenamine	$\overline{X}$	average of all X's
914	neoarsphenamine	α	alpha particle is proportional to
℞	take	$\neq$	does not equal
6-MP	6-mercaptopurine	>	greater than
^{3}HT	H$_3$T, triated thymidine	<	less than
2d	second	χ^2	chi square (test)
2°	secondary	σ	1/1000 of a second standard deviation
2ndry	secondary		
2×	twice	℈	scruple
×2	twice	℥	ounce
1×	once	f℥	fluid ounce

μ	micron	μu	microunit
$\mu\mu$	micromicron	μv	microvolt
μc	microcurie	μw	microwatt
μEq	microequivalent	μV	milligamma (micromicrogram, picogram)
μf	microfarad		
μg	microgram	mμc	millimicrocurie (nanocurie)
μl	microliter		
$\mu\mu$c	micromicrocurie (picocurie)	mμg	millimicrogram (nanogram)
$\mu\mu$g	micromicrogram (picogram)	mμ	millimicron
		ℨ	drachm dram
μM	micromolar		
μr	microroentgen	f ℨ	fluidrachm fluidram
μsec	microsecond